Practice the TEAS®!

Test of Essential Academic Skills

Practice Test Questions

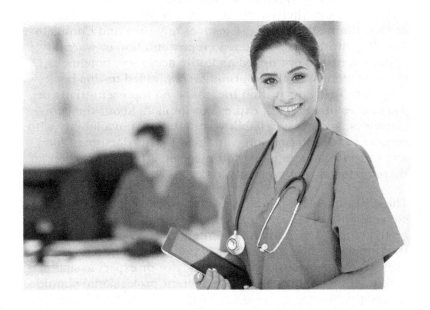

Published by

Complete **TEST** Preparation Inc.

Practice the TEAS®!

We strongly recommend that students check with exam providers for up-to-date information regarding test content.

ISBN-13: 978-1928077756 (Complete Test Preparation Inc.)

ISBN-10: 1928077757

Version 7.5 April 2018

Published by
Complete Test Preparation Inc.
Victoria BC Canada
Visit us on the web at http://www.test-preparation.ca
Printed in the USA

About Complete Test Preparation Inc.

The Complete Test Preparation Team has been publishing high quality study materials since 2005. Over 1 million students visit our websites every year, and thousands of students, teachers and parents all over the world (over 100 countries) have purchased our teaching materials, curriculum, study guides and practice tests.

Complete Test Preparation is committed to providing students with the best study materials and practice tests available on the market. Members of our team combine years of teaching experience, with experienced writers and editors, all with advanced degrees.

Feedback

We welcome your feedback. Email us at feedback@test-preparation.ca with your comments and suggestions. We carefully review all suggestions and often incorporate reader suggestions into upcoming versions. As a Print on Demand Publisher, we update our products frequently.

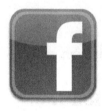 **Find us on Facebook**

Contents

Getting Started

CONGRATULATIONS! By deciding to take the Test of Essential Academic Skills (TEAS® V) Exam, you have taken the first step toward a great future! Of course, there is no point in taking this important examination unless you intend to do your best to earn the highest grade you possibly can. That means getting yourself organized and discovering the best approaches, methods and strategies to master the material. Yes, that will require real effort and dedication on your part, but if you are willing to focus your energy and devote the study time necessary, before you know it you will be opening that letter of acceptance to the school of your dreams.

We know that taking on a new endeavour can be a little scary, and it is easy to feel unsure of where to begin. That's where we come in. This study guide is designed to help you improve your test-taking skills, show you a few tricks of the trade and increase both your competency and confidence.

The Test of Essential Academic Skills Exam

Content areas for the TEAS® V are: Reading, Math, Science and English.

Reading
Paragraph Comprehension
Passage Comprehension

Mathematics
Numbers and Operations
Algebraic Applications
Data Interpretation
Measurement
Metric Conversion

Science
Human Body Science
Life Science
Earth and Physical Science
Scientific Reasoning

English and Language Usage
English Grammar and Usage
Word meaning in Context
Spelling and Punctuation
Sentence Structure

While we seek to make our guide as comprehensive as possible, note that like all entrance exams, the TEAS® V Exam might be adjusted at some future point. New material might be added, or content that is no longer relevant or applicable might be removed. It is always a good idea to give the materials you receive when you register to take the TEAS® a careful review.

It is also important to note that not all schools use all of the modules or the same version. Make sure you know which version of the TEAS and which modules your school will be using so you do not waste valuable study time studying material that is no on your school's test!

The TEAS® Study Plan

Now that you have made the decision to take the TEAS, it is time to get started. Before you do another thing, you will need to figure out a plan of attack. The very best study tip is to start early! The longer the time period you devote to regular study practice, the more likely you will be to retain the material and be able to access it quickly. If you thought that 1x20 is the same as 2x10, guess what? It really is not, when it comes to study time. Reviewing material for just an hour per day over the course of 20 days is far better than studying for two hours a day for only 10 days. The more often you revisit a particular piece of information, the better you will know it. Not only will your grasp and understanding be better, but your ability to reach into your brain and quickly and efficiently pull out the tidbit you need, will be greatly enhanced as well.

The great Chinese scholar and philosopher Confucius believed that true knowledge could be defined as knowing both what you know and what you do not know. The first step in preparing for the TEAS® Exam is to assess your strengths and weaknesses. You may already have an idea of what you know and what you do not know, but evaluating yourself using our Self-Assessment modules for each of the three areas, math, english science and reading, will clarify the details.

Making a Study Schedule

In order to make your study time most productive you will need to develop a study plan. The purpose of the plan is to organize all the bits of pieces of information in such a way that you will not feel overwhelmed. Rome was not built in a day, and learning everything you will need to know to pass the TEAS® Exam is going to take time, too. Arranging the material you need to learn into manageable chunks is the best way to go. Each study session should make you feel as though you have succeeded in accomplishing your goal, and your goal is simply to learn what you planned to learn during that particular session. Try to organize the content in such a way that each study session builds on previous ones. That way, you will retain the information, be better able to access it, and review the previous bits and pieces at the same time.

Self-assessment

The Best Study Tip! The very best study tip is to start early! The longer you study regularly, the more you will retain and 'learn' the material. Studying for 1 hour per day for 20 days is far better than studying for 2 hours for 10 days.

What don't you know?

The first step is to assess your strengths and weaknesses.

You may already have an idea of where your weaknesses are, or you can take our Self-assessment modules for each of the areas, math, English, science and reading.

Below is a table to assess your exam readiness in each content area. You can fill this in now, and correct if necessary after completing the self-assessments, or fill it in after you have taken the self-assessments.

Exam Readiness Assessment

Exam Component	Rate 1 to 5
Reading	
Paragraph Comprehension	
Passage Comprehension	
English	
Grammar Word Meaning (Vocabulary - Meaning in Context) Spelling & Punctuation Sentence Structure	
Math	
Basic Math	
Algebra	
Data Interpretation	
Measurement	
Science	
Human Body Science (Anatomy and Physiology)	
Life Science (Biology, Ecology etc.)	
Earth and Physical Sciences	
Scientific Reasoning	

Making a Study Schedule

The key to making a study plan is to divide the material you need to learn into manageable size and learn it, while at the same time reviewing the material that you already know.

Using the table above, any scores of 3 or below, you need to spend time learning, going over and practicing this subject area. A score of 4 means you need to review the material, but you don't have to spend time re-learning. A score of 5 and you are OK with just an occasional review before the exam.

A score of 0 or 1 means you really need to work on this area and should allocate the most time and the highest priority. Some students prefer a 5-day plan and others a 10-day plan. It also depends on how much time you have until the exam.

Here is an example of a 5-day plan based on an example from the table above:

Basic Math: 1 Study 1 hour everyday – review on last day
Life Science: 3 Study 1 hour for 2 days then ½ hour a day, then review
Vocabulary: 4 Review every second day
Spelling: 2 Study 1 hour on the first day – then ½ hour everyday
Reading: 5 Review for ½ hour every other day
Algebra: 5 Review for ½ hour every other day
Human Body Science: 5 very confident – review a few times.

Using this example, here is a sample study plan which you can adapt to your own situation:

Day	Subject	Time
Monday		
Study	Basic Math	1 hour
Study	Spelling	1 hour
½ hour break		
Study	Life Sciences	1 hour
Review	Human Body Sciences	½ hour
Tuesday		
Study	Basic Math	1 hour
Study	Spelling	½ hour
½ hour break		
Study	Data Interpretation	½ hour
Review	Vocabulary	½ hour
Review	Grammar	½ hour
Wednesday		
Study	Basic Math	1 hour
Study	Spelling	½ hour
½ hour break		
Study	LIfe Sciences	½ hour
Review	Human Body Sciences	½ hour
Thursday		
Study	Basic Math	½ hour
Study	Spelling	½ hour
Review	Life Sciences	½ hour
½ hour break		
Review	Grammar	½ hour
Review	Vocabulary	½ hour
Friday		
Review	Basic Math	½ hour
Review	Spelling	½ hour
Review	Life Sciences	½ hour
½ hour break		
Review	Vocabulary	½ hour
Review	Grammar	½ hour

Practice Test Questions Set 1

Section I – Reading

Questions: 30
Time: 30 Minutes

Section II – Mathematics

Questions: 30
Time: 30 Minutes

Section III – English and Language Usage

Questions: 30
Time: 30 Minutes

Section IV –Science

Questions: 48
Time: 40 minutes

The questions below are not the same as you will find on the TEAS® - that would be too easy! And nobody knows what the questions will be and they change all the time. Below are general questions that cover the same subject areas as the TEAS®. So, while the format and exact wording of the questions may differ slightly, and change from year to year, if you can answer the questions below, you will have no problem with the TEAS®.

For the best results, take these practice test questions as if it were the real exam. Set aside time when you will not be disturbed, and a location that is quiet and free of distractions. Read the instructions carefully, read each question carefully, and answer to the best of your ability.

Use the bubble answer sheets provided. When you have completed the practice questions, check your answer against the Answer Key and read the explanation provided.

You are given 209 minutes to complete the full TEAS® exam.

Do not attempt more than one set of practice test questions in one day. After completing the first practice test, wait two or three days before attempting the second set of questions.

Section 1 - Reading

	A B C D E		A B C D E
1	○○○○○	21	○○○○○
2	○○○○○	22	○○○○○
3	○○○○○	23	○○○○○
4	○○○○○	24	○○○○○
5	○○○○○	25	○○○○○
6	○○○○○	26	○○○○○
7	○○○○○	27	○○○○○
8	○○○○○	28	○○○○○
9	○○○○○	29	○○○○○
10	○○○○○	30	○○○○○
11	○○○○○	31	○○○○○
12	○○○○○	32	○○○○○
13	○○○○○	33	○○○○○
14	○○○○○	34	○○○○○
15	○○○○○	35	○○○○○
16	○○○○○		
17	○○○○○		
18	○○○○○		
19	○○○○○		
20	○○○○○		

Section II - Math

A B C D E   A B C D E

1 ○○○○○   21 ○○○○○
2 ○○○○○   22 ○○○○○
3 ○○○○○   23 ○○○○○
4 ○○○○○   24 ○○○○○
5 ○○○○○   25 ○○○○○
6 ○○○○○   26 ○○○○○
7 ○○○○○   27 ○○○○○
8 ○○○○○   28 ○○○○○
9 ○○○○○   29 ○○○○○
10 ○○○○○ 30 ○○○○○
11 ○○○○○
12 ○○○○○
13 ○○○○○
14 ○○○○○
15 ○○○○○
16 ○○○○○
17 ○○○○○
18 ○○○○○
19 ○○○○○
20 ○○○○○

Section III English

	A	B	C	D	E			A	B	C	D	E
1	○	○	○	○	○		21	○	○	○	○	○
2	○	○	○	○	○		22	○	○	○	○	○
3	○	○	○	○	○		23	○	○	○	○	○
4	○	○	○	○	○		24	○	○	○	○	○
5	○	○	○	○	○		25	○	○	○	○	○
6	○	○	○	○	○		26	○	○	○	○	○
7	○	○	○	○	○		27	○	○	○	○	○
8	○	○	○	○	○		28	○	○	○	○	○
9	○	○	○	○	○		29	○	○	○	○	○
10	○	○	○	○	○		30	○	○	○	○	○
11	○	○	○	○	○							
12	○	○	○	○	○							
13	○	○	○	○	○							
14	○	○	○	○	○							
15	○	○	○	○	○							
16	○	○	○	○	○							
17	○	○	○	○	○							
18	○	○	○	○	○							
19	○	○	○	○	○							
20	○	○	○	○	○							

Section IV – Science

	A B C D E		A B C D E
1	○○○○○	26	○○○○○
2	○○○○○	27	○○○○○
3	○○○○○	28	○○○○○
4	○○○○○	29	○○○○○
5	○○○○○	30	○○○○○
6	○○○○○	31	○○○○○
7	○○○○○	32	○○○○○
8	○○○○○	33	○○○○○
9	○○○○○	34	○○○○○
10	○○○○○	35	○○○○○
11	○○○○○	36	○○○○○
12	○○○○○	37	○○○○○
13	○○○○○	38	○○○○○
14	○○○○○	39	○○○○○
15	○○○○○	40	○○○○○
16	○○○○○	41	○○○○○
17	○○○○○	42	○○○○○
18	○○○○○	43	○○○○○
19	○○○○○	44	○○○○○
20	○○○○○	45	○○○○○
21	○○○○○	46	○○○○○
22	○○○○○	47	○○○○○
23	○○○○○	48	○○○○○
24	○○○○○	49	○○○○○
25	○○○○○	50	○○○○○

Directions: The following questions are based on several reading passages. Each passage is followed by a series of questions. Read each passage carefully, and then answer the questions based on it. You may reread the passage as often as you wish. When you have finished answering the questions based on one passage, go right onto the next passage. Choose the best answer based on the information given and implied.

Questions 1 – 4 refer to the following passage.

Passage 1 - The Life of Helen Keller

Many people have heard of Helen Keller. She is famous because she was unable to see or hear, but learned to speak and read and went onto attend college and earn a degree. Her life is a very interesting story, one that she developed into an autobiography, which was then adapted into both a stage play and a movie. How did Helen Keller overcome her disabilities to become a famous woman? Read onto find out. Helen Keller was not born blind and deaf. When she was a small baby, she had a very high fever for several days. As a result of her sudden illness, baby Helen lost her eyesight and her hearing. Because she was so young when she went deaf and blind, Helen Keller never had any recollection of being able to see or hear. Since she could not hear, she could not learn to talk. Since she could not see, it was difficult for her to move around. For the first six years of her life, her world was very still and dark.

Imagine what Helen's childhood must have been like. She could not hear her mother's voice. She could not see the beauty of her parent's farm. She could not recognize who was giving her a hug, or a bath or even where her bedroom was each night. More sad, she could not communicate with her parents in any way. She could not express her feelings or tell them the things she wanted. It must have been a very sad childhood.

When Helen was six years old, her parents hired her a teacher named Anne Sullivan. Anne was a young woman who was almost blind. However, she could hear and she could read

Braille, so she was a perfect teacher for young Helen. At first, Anne had a very hard time teaching Helen anything. She described her first impression of Helen as a "wild thing, not a child." Helen did not like Anne at first either. She bit and hit Anne when Anne tried to teach her. However, the two of them eventually came to have a great deal of love and respect.

Anne taught Helen to hear by putting her hands on people's throats. She could feel the sounds that people made. In time, Helen learned to feel what people said. Next, Anne taught Helen to read Braille, which is a way that books are written for the blind. Finally, Anne taught Helen to talk. Although Helen did learn to talk, it was hard for anyone but Anne to understand her.

As Helen grew older, more and more people were amazed by her story. She went to college and wrote books about her life. She gave talks to the public, with Anne at her side, translating her words. Today, both Anne Sullivan and Helen Keller are famous women who are respected for their lives' work.

1. Helen Keller could not see and hear and so, what was her biggest problem in childhood?

    a. Inability to communicate

    b. Inability to walk

    c. Inability to play

    d. Inability to eat

2. Helen learned to hear by feeling the vibrations people made when they spoke. What were these vibrations were felt through?

    a. Mouth

    b. Throat

    c. Ears

    d. Lips

3. From the passage, we can infer that Anne Sullivan was a patient teacher. We can infer this because

   a. Helen hit and bit her and Anne still remained her teacher.

   b. Anne taught Helen to read only.

   c. Anne was hard of hearing too.

   d. Anne wanted to be a teacher.

4. Helen Keller learned to speak but Anne translated her words when she spoke in public. The reason Helen needed a translator was because

   a. Helen spoke another language.

   b. Helen's words were hard for people to understand.

   c. Helen spoke very quietly.

   d. Helen did not speak but only used sign language.

Questions 5 – 8 refer to the following passage.

Passage 2 - Ways Characters Communicate in Theater

Playwrights give their characters voices in a way that gives depth and added meaning to what happens on stage during their play. There are different types of speech in scripts that allow characters to talk with themselves, with other characters, and even with the audience.

It is very unique to theater that characters may talk "to themselves." When characters do this, the speech they give is called a soliloquy. Soliloquies are usually poetic, introspective, moving, and can tell audience members about the feelings, motivations, or suspicions of an individual character without that character having to reveal them to other characters on stage. "To be or not to be" is a famous soliloquy given by Hamlet as he considers difficult but important themes, such as life and death.

The most common type of communication in plays is when one character is speaking to another or a group of other characters. This is generally called dialogue, but can also be called monologue if one character speaks without being interrupted for a long time. It is not necessarily the most important type of communication, but it is the most common because the plot of the play cannot really progress without it.

Lastly, and most unique to theater (although it has been used somewhat in film) is when a character speaks directly to the audience. This is called an aside, and scripts usually specifically direct actors to do this. Asides are usually comical, an inside joke between the character and the audience, and very short. The actor will usually face the audience when delivering them, even if it's for a moment, so the audience can recognize this move as an aside.

All three of these types of communication are important to the art of theater, and have been perfected by famous playwrights like Shakespeare. Understanding these types of communication can help an audience member grasp what is artful about the script and action of a play.

5. According to the passage, characters in plays communicate to

    a. move the plot forward

    b. show the private thoughts and feelings of one character

    c. make the audience laugh

    d. add beauty and artistry to the play

6. When Hamlet delivers "To be or not to be," he can most likely be described as

    a. solitary

    b. thoughtful

    c. dramatic

    d. hopeless

7. The author uses parentheses to punctuate "although it has been used somewhat in film,"

> a. to show that films are less important
>
> b. instead of using commas so that the sentence is not interrupted
>
> c. because parenthesis help separate details that are not as important
>
> d. to show that films are not as artistic

Questions 9 – 11 refer to the following passage.

Passage 3 - Low Blood Sugar

As the name suggest, low blood sugar is low sugar levels in the bloodstream. This can occur when you have not eaten properly and undertake strenuous activity, or, when you are very hungry. When Low blood sugar occurs regularly and is ongoing, it is a medical condition called hypoglycemia. This condition can occur in diabetics and in healthy adults.

Causes of low blood sugar can include excessive alcohol consumption, metabolic problems, stomach surgery, pancreas, liver or kidneys problems, as well as a side-effect of some medications.

Symptoms

There are different symptoms depending on the severity of the case.

Mild hypoglycemia can lead to feelings of nausea and hunger. The patient may also feel nervous, jittery and have fast heart beats. Sweaty skin, clammy and cold skin are likely symptoms.
Moderate hypoglycemia can result in a short temper, confusion, nervousness, fear and blurring of vision. The patient may feel weak and unsteady.

Severe cases of hypoglycemia can lead to seizures, coma,

fainting spells, nightmares, headaches, excessive sweats and severe tiredness.

Diagnosis of low blood sugar

A doctor can diagnosis this medical condition by asking the patient questions and testing blood and urine samples. Home testing kits are available for patients to monitor blood sugar levels. It is important to see a qualified doctor though. The doctor can administer tests to ensure that will safely rule out other medical conditions that could affect blood sugar levels.

Treatment

Quick treatments include drinking or eating foods and drinks with high sugar contents. Good examples include soda, fruit juice, hard candy and raisins. Glucose energy tablets can also help. Doctors may also recommend medications and well as changes in diet and exercise routine to treat chronic low blood sugar.

8. Based on the article, which of the following is true?

a. Low blood sugar can happen to anyone.

b. Low blood sugar only happens to diabetics.

c. Low blood sugar can occur even.

d. None of the statements are true.

9. Which of the following are the author's opinion?

a. Quick treatments include drinking or eating foods and drinks with high sugar contents.

b. None of the statements are opinions.

c. This condition can occur in diabetics and also in healthy adults.

d. There are different symptoms depending on the severity of the case

10. What is the author's purpose?

   a. To inform

   b. To persuade

   c. To entertain

   d. To analyze

11. Which of the following is not a detail?

   a. A doctor can diagnosis this medical condition by asking the patient questions and testing.

   b. A doctor will test blood and urine samples.

   c. Glucose energy tablets can also help.

   d. Home test kits monitor blood sugar levels.

Questions 12 – 14 refer to the following passage.

How To Get A Good Nights Sleep

Sleep is just as essential for healthy living as water, air and food. Sleep allows the body to rest and replenish depleted energy levels. Sometimes we may for various reasons experience difficulty sleeping which has a serious effect on our health. Those who have prolonged sleeping problems are facing a serious medical condition and should see a qualified doctor when possible for help. Here is simple guide that can help you sleep better at night.

Try to create a natural pattern of waking up and sleeping around the same time everyday. This means avoiding going to bed too early and oversleeping past your usual wake up time. Going to bed and getting up at radically different times everyday confuses your body clock. Try to establish a natural rhythm as much as you can.

Exercises and a bit of physical activity can help you sleep better at night. If you are having problem sleeping, try to be as active as you can during the day. If you are tired from physical activity, falling asleep is a natural and easy process for your body. If you remain inactive during the day, you will find it harder to sleep properly at night. Try walking, jogging, swimming or simple stretches as you get close to your bed time.

Afternoon naps are great to refresh you during the day, but they may also keep you awake at night. If you feel sleepy during the day, get up, take a walk and get busy to keep from sleeping. Stretching is a good way to increase blood flow to the brain and keep you alert so that you don't sleep during the day. This will help you sleep better night.

> A warm bath or a glass of milk in the evening can help your body relax and prepare for sleep. A cold bath will wake you up and keep you up for several hours. Also avoid eating too late before bed.

12. How would you describe this sentence?

a. A recommendation

b. An opinion

c. A fact

d. A diagnosis

13. Which of the following is an alternative title for this article?

a. Exercise and a good night's sleep

b. Benefits of a good night's sleep

c. Tips for a good night's sleep

d. Lack of sleep is a serious medical condition

14. Which of the following cannot be inferred from this article?

a. Biking is helpful for getting a good night's sleep

b. Mental activity is helpful for getting a good night's sleep

c. Eating bedtime snacks is not recommended

d. Getting up at the same time is helpful for a good night's sleep

15. What is a disadvantage of taking naps?

a. They may keep you awake.

b. There are no disadvantages

c. They may help you sleep better

d. They may affect your diet

Question 16 refers to the following Table of Contents.

Contents

Contents

16. Consider the table of contents above. What page would you find information about natural selection and adaptation?

    a. 81

    b. 90

    c. 110

    d. 132

Questions 17 – 19 refer to the following passage.

Passage 5 - Pearl Harbor

A Day That Will Live in Infamy! Attack on Pearl Harbor
In 1941, the world was at war. The United States was trying very hard to keep itself out of the conflict. In Europe, the countries of Germany and Italy had formed an alliance to expand their land and territory. Germany had already taken over Poland, Denmark, and parts of France. They were heading next toward England and due to all the fighting in Europe, there were battles taking place as far south as North Africa, where the German and Italian armies were fighting the British.

This got even worse when the Asian nation of Japan formed an alliance with Germany and Italy. Together, the three countries called themselves, the AXIS. Now, the war was in the Pacific as well as in Europe and Northern Africa. A great deal of Americans felt that perhaps now was the time for the United States to join with its ally, Great Britain and stop the Axis from taking over more regions of the world.

In 1941, Franklin Roosevelt was President of the United States. His fear at the time was that Japan would try to take over many countries in Asia. He did not want to see that happen, so he moved some of the United States warships that had been stationed in San Diego, to the military base at Pearl Harbor, in Honolulu, Hawaii.

Japan quietly plotted their attack. They waited until the

early hours of the morning on Sunday, December 7, 1941. Then, 350 Japanese war plans began to drop bombs on the U.S. ships at Pearl Harbor. The first bombs fell at 7:48 am and a mere 90 minutes later, the attack was over. Pearl Harbor was decimated. 8 battleships were damaged. Eleven ships were sunk and 300 U.S. planes were destroyed. Most devastating was the loss of life 2,400 U.S. military members was killed in the attack and 1, 282 were injured.

President Roosevelt addressed the country via the radio and said "Today is a day that will live in infamy." He asked Congress to declare war on Japan. War was declared on Japan on December 8th and on Germany and Italy on December 11th. The United States had entered World War Two.

17. After reading the passage, what can you infer infamy means?

a. Famous

b. Remembered in a good way

c. Remembered in a bad way

d. Easily forgotten

18. What three countries formed the Axis?

a. Italy, England, Germany

b. United States, England, Italy

c. Germany, Japan, Italy

d. Germany, Japan, United States

19. What do you think was President Roosevelt's reason for moving warships to Pearl Harbor?

a. He feared Japan would bomb San Diego

b. He knew Japan was going to attack Pearl Harbor

c. He was planning to attack Japan

d. He wanted to try and protect Asian countries from Japanese takeover

20. Why do you think Japan chose a Sunday morning at 7:48 am for their attack?

    a. They knew the military slept late

    b. There is a law against bombing countries on a Sunday

    c. They wanted the attack to catch people by surprise

    d. That was the only free time they had to attack.

Questions 21 - 24 refer to the following recipe.

If You Have Allergies, You're Not Alone

People who experience allergies might joke that their immune systems have let them down or are seriously lacking. Truthfully though, people who experience allergic reactions or allergy symptoms during certain times of the year have heightened immune systems that are, "better" than those of people who have perfectly healthy but less militant immune systems.

Still, when a person has an allergic reaction, they are having an adverse reaction to a substance that is considered normal to most people. Mild allergic reactions usually have symptoms like itching, runny nose, red eyes, or bumps or discoloration of the skin. More serious allergic reactions, such as those to animal and insect poisons or certain foods, may result in the closing of the throat, swelling of the eyes, low blood pressure, inability to breath, and can even be fatal.

Different treatments help different allergies, and which one a person uses depends on the nature and severity of the allergy. It is recommended to patients with severe allergies to take extra precautions, such as carrying an EpiPen, which treats anaphylactic shock and may prevent death, always in order for the remedy to be readily available and more effective. When an allergy is not so severe, treatments may be used just relieve a person of uncomfortable symptoms. Over the counter allergy medicines treat milder symptoms, and can be bought at any grocery store and used in moderation to help people with allergies live normally.

There are many tests available to assess whether a person has allergies or what they may be allergic to, and advances in these tests and the medicine used to treat patients continues to improve. Despite this fact, allergies still affect many people throughout the year or even every day. Medicines used to treat allergies have side effects of their own, and it is difficult to bring the body into balance with the use of medicine. Regardless, many of those who live with allergies are grateful for what is available and find it useful in maintaining their lifestyles.

21. According to this passage, it can be understood that the word "militant" belongs in a group with the words:

    a. sickly, ailing, faint

    b. strength, power, vigor

    c. active, fighting, warring

    d. worn, tired, breaking down

22. The author says that "medicines used to treat allergies have side-effects of their own" to

    a. point out that doctors aren't very good at diagnosing and treating allergies

    b. argue that because of the large number of people with allergies, a cure will never be found

    c. explain that allergy medicines aren't cures and some compromise must be made

    d. argue that more wholesome remedies should be researched and medicines banned

23. It can be inferred that _____ recommend that some people with allergies carry medicine with them.

    a. the author

    b. doctors

    c. the makers of EpiPen

    d. people with allergies

24. The author has written this passage to

  a. inform readers on symptoms of allergies so people with allergies can get help

  b. persuade readers to be proud of having allergies

  c. inform readers on different remedies so people with allergies receive the right help

  d. describe different types of allergies, their symptoms, and their remedies

Questions 25 – 26 refer to the following email.

SUBJECT: MEDICAL STAFF CHANGES

To all staff:

This email is to advise you of a paper on recommended medical staff changes has been posted to the Human Resources website.

The contents are of primary interest to medical staff, other staff may be interested in reading it, particularly those in medical support roles.

The paper deals with several major issues:

  1. Improving our ability to attract top quality staff to the hospital, and retain our existing staff. These changes will make our position and departmental names internationally recognizable and comparable with North American and North Asian departments and positions.

  2. Improving our ability to attract top quality staff by introducing greater flexibility in the departmental structure.

  3. General comments on issues to be further discussed in relation to research staff.

The changes outlined in this paper are significant. I encourage you to read the document and send to me any comments you may have, so that it can be enhanced and improved.

Gordon Simms
Administrator,
Seven Oaks Regional Hospital

25. Are all hospital staff required to read the document posted to the Human Resources website?

  a. Yes all staff are required to read the document.

  b. No, reading the document is optional.

  c. Only medical staff are required to read the document.

  d. none of the above are correct.

26. Have the changes to medical staff been made?

  a. Yes, the changes have been made.

  b. No, the changes are only being discussed.

  c. Some of the changes have been made.

  d. None of the choices are correct.

Questions 27 – 30 refer to the following passage.

When a Poet Longs to Mourn, He Writes an Elegy

Poems are an expressive, especially emotional, form of writing. They have been present in literature virtually from the time civilizations invented the written word. Poets often portrayed as moody, secluded, and even troubled, but this is because poets are introspective and feel deeply about the current events and cultural norms they are surrounded with. Poets often produce the most telling literature, giving insight into the society and mind-set they come from. This can be done in many forms.

The oldest types of poems often include many stanzas, may or may not rhyme, and are more about telling a story than experimenting with language or words. The most common types of ancient poetry are epics, which are usually extremely long stories that follow a hero through his journey, or ellegies, which are often solemn in tone and used to mourn or lament something or someone. The Mesopotamians are often said to have invented the written word, and their literature is among the oldest in the world, including the epic poem titled "Epic of Gilgamesh." Similar in style and length to "Gilgamesh" is "Beowulf," an ellegy written in Old English and set in Scandinavia. These poems are often used by professors as the earliest examples of literature.

The importance of poetry was revived in the Renaissance. At this time, Europeans discovered the style and beauty of ancient Greek arts, and poetry was among those. Shakespeare is the most well-known poet of the time, and he used poetry not only to write poems but also to write plays for the theater. The most popular forms of poetry during the Renaissance included villanelles, (a nineteen-line poetic form) sonnets, as well as the epic. Poets during this time focused on style and form, and developed very specific rules and outlines for how an exceptional poem should be written.

As often happens in the arts, modern poets have rejected the constricting rules of Renaissance poets, and free form poems are much more popular. Some modern poems would read just like stories if they weren't arranged into lines and stanzas. It is difficult to tell which poems and poets will be the most important, because works of art often become more famous in hindsight, after the poet has died and society can look at itself without being in the moment. Modern poetry continues to develop, and will no doubt continue to change as values, thought, and writing continue to change.

Poems can be among the most enlightening and uplifting texts for a person to read if they are looking to connect with the past, connect with other people, or try to gain an understanding of what is happening in their time.

27. In summary, the author has written this passage

a. as a foreword that will introduce a poem in a book or magazine

b. because she loves poetry and wants more people to like it

c. to give a brief history of poems

d. to convince students to write poems

28. The author organizes the paragraphs mainly by

a. moving chronologically, explaining which types of poetry were common in that time

b. talking about new types of poems each paragraph and explaining them a little

c. focusing on one poet or group of people and the poems they wrote

d. explaining older types of poetry so she can talk about modern poetry

29. The author's claim that poetry has been around "virtually from the time civilizations invented the written word" is supported by the detail that

a. Beowulf is written in Old English, which is not really in use any longer

b. epic poems told stories about heroes

c. the Renaissance poets tried to copy Greek poets

d. the Mesopotamians are credited with both inventing the word and writing "Epic of Gilgamesh"

30. According to the passage, it can be understood that the word "telling" means

a. speaking

b. significant

c. soothing

d. wordy

Questions 31 – 32 refer to the following passage.

Scottish Wind Farms

The Scottish Government has a targeted plan of generating 100% of Scotland's electricity through renewable energy by 2020. Renewable energy sources include sun, water and wind power. Scotland uses all forms but its fastest growing energy is wind energy. Wind power is generated through the use of wind turbines, placed onshore and offshore. Wind turbines that are grouped together in large numbers are called wind farms. A majority of Scottish citizens say that the wind farms are necessary to meet current and future energy needs, and would like to see an increase in the number of wind farms. They cite the fact that wind energy does not cause pollution, there are low operational costs, and most importantly due to the definition of renewable energy it cannot be depleted.

31. What is Scotland's fastest growing source of renewable energy?

    a. Solar Panels

    b. Hydroelectric

    c. Wind

    d. Fossil Fuels

32. Why do the majority of Scottish citizens agree with the Government's plan?

    a. Their concern for current and future energy needs

    b. Because of the low operational costs

    c. Because they are out of sight

    d. Because it provides jobs

Questions 33 – 34 refer to the following passage.

Scottish Wind Farms II

However, there is still a public debate concerning the use of wind farms to generate energy. The most cited argument against wind energy is that the upfront investment is expensive. They also argue that it is aesthetically displeasing, they are noisy, and they create a serious threat to wildlife in the area. While wind energy is renewable, or cannot be depleted, it does not mean that wind is always available. Wind is fluctuating, or intermittent, and therefore not suited to meet the base amount of energy demand, meaning if there is no wind then no energy is being created.

33. What is the biggest argument against wind energy?

   a. The turbines are noisy

   b. The turbines endanger wildlife

   c. The turbines are expensive to build

   d. They are aesthetically displeasing

34. What is the best way to describe this article's description of wind energy?

   a. Loud and ever present

   b. The cheapest form of renewable energy

   c. The only source of renewable energy in Scotland

   d. Clean and renewable but fluctuating

Save the Children

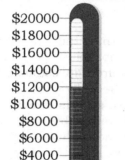

35. Consider the graphic above. The Save the Children fund has a fund-raising goal of $20,000. Approximately how much of their goal have they achieved?

    a. 3/5

    b. 3/4

    c. 1/2

    d. 1/3

Section II – Math

1. What is 1/3 of 3/4?

    a. 1/4

    b. 1/3

    c. 2/3

    d. 3/4

2. Susan wants to buy a leather jacket that costs $545.00 and is on sale for 10% off. What is the approximate cost?

    a. $525

    b. $450

    c. $475

    d. $500

3. 3.14 + 2.73 + 23.7 =

    a. 28.57

    b. 30.57

    c. 29.56

    d. 29.57

4. A woman spent 15% of her income on an item and ends with $120. What percentage of her income is left?

    a. 12%

    b. 85%

    c. 75%

    d. 95%

5. Express 0.27 + 0.33 as a fraction.

    a. 3/6

    b. 4/7

    c. 3/5

    d. 2/7

6. 8 is what percent of 40?

    a. 10%

    b. 15%

    c. 20%

    d. 25%

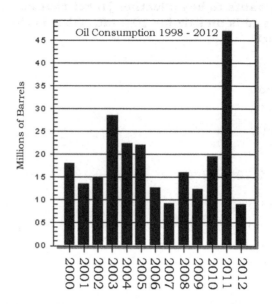

7. The graph above shows oil consumption in millions of barrels for the period, 1998 - 2012. What year did oil consumption peak?

    a. 2011
    b. 2010
    c. 2008
    d. 2009

8. Translate the following into an equation: 2 + a number divided by 7.

    a. $(2 + X)/7$
    b. $(7 + X)/2$
    c. $(2 + 7)/X$
    d. $2/(7 + X)$

9. .4% of 36 is

   a. 1.44

   b. .144

   c. 14.4

   d. 144

10. The physician ordered 5 mg Coumadin; 10 mg/tablet is on hand. How many tablets will you give?

   a. .5 tablet

   b. 1 tablet

   c. .75 tablet

   d. 1.5 tablets

11. The physician ordered 20 mg Tylenol/kg of body weight; on hand is 80 mg/tablet. The child weighs 12 kg. How many tablets will you give?

   a. 1 tablet

   b. 3 tablets

   c. 2 tablets

   d. 4 tablets

12. Consider the following population growth chart.

Country	Population 2000	Population 2005
Japan	122,251,000	128,057,000
China	1,145,195,000	1,341,335,000
United States	253,339,000	310,384,000
Indonesia	184,346,000	239,871,000

What country is growing the fastest?

 a. Japan

 b. China

 c. United States

 d. Indonesia

13. If y = 4 and x = 3, solve yx^3

 a. -108

 b. 108

 c. 27

 d. 4

14. What number is MCMXC?

 a. 1990

 b. 1980

 c. 2000

 d. 1995

15. Convert 16 quarts to gallons.

 a. 1 gallons

 b. 8 gallons

 c. 4 gallons

 d. 4.5 gallons

16. Convert 45 kg. to pounds.

 a. 10 pounds

 b. 100 pounds

 c. 1,000 pounds

 d. 110 pounds

17. Translate the following into an equation: three plus a number times 7 equals 42.

    a. $7(3 + X) = 42$

    b. $3(X + 7) = 42$

    c. $3X + 7 = 42$

    d. $(3 + 7)X = 42$

18. In a class of 83 students, 72 are present. What percent of the students are absent? Provide answer up to two significant digits.

    a. 12%

    b. 13%

    c. 14%

    d. 15%

19. $5x+2(x+7) = 14x - 7$. Find x

    a. 1

    b. 2

    c. 3

    d. 4

20. $5(z+1) = 3(z+2) + 11$. Find z

    a. 2

    b. 4

    c. 6

    d. 12

21. The price of a book went from $20 to $25. What percent did the price increase?

   a. 5%

   b. 10%

   c. 20%

   d. 25%

22. A boy is given 2 apples while his sister is given 8 oranges. What is the ratio between the boy's apples and her oranges?

   a. 1:2

   b. 2:4

   c. 1:4

   d. 2:1

23. In the time required to serve 43 customers, a server breaks 2 glasses and slips 5 times. The next day, the same server breaks 10 glasses. Assuming that glasses broken is proportional to customers served, how many customers did she serve?

   a. 25

   b. 43

   c. 86

   d. 215

24. A square lawn has an area of 62,500 square meters. What is the cost of building fence around it at a rate of $5.5 per meter?

   a. $4000

   b. $4500

   c. $5000

   d. $5500

25. Solve for n, when 5n + (19 – 2) = 67.

    a. 21

    b. 10

    c. 15

    d. 7

26. Below is the attendance for a class of 45.

Day	Absent Students
Monday	5
Tuesday	9
Wednesday	4
Thursday	10
Friday	6

What is the average attendance for the week?

    a. 88%

    b. 85%

    c. 81%

    d. 77%

27. A distributor purchased 550 kilograms of potatoes for $165. He distributed these at a rate of $6.4 per 20 kilograms to 15 shops, $3.4 per 10 kilograms to 12 shops and the remainder at $1.8 per 5 kilograms. If his total distribution cost is $10, what will his profit be?

    a. $10.40

    b. $8.60

    c. $14.90

    d. $23.40

28. How much pay does Mr. Johnson receive if he gives half of his pay to his family, $250 to his landlord, and has exactly 3/7 of his pay left over?

    a. $3600

    b. $3500

    c. $2800

    d. $1750

29. A boy has 4 red, 5 green and 2 yellow balls. He chooses two balls randomly. What is the probability that one is red and other is green?

    a. 2/11

    b. 19/22

    c. 20/121

    d. 9/11

30. The cost of waterproofing canvas is .50 a square yard. What's the total cost for waterproofing a canvas truck cover that is 15' x 24'?

    a. $18.00

    b. $6.67

    c. $180.00

    d. $20.00

Section III - English

1. Choose the sentence with the correct grammar.

    a. Don would never have thought of that book, but you could have reminded him.

    b. Don would never of thought of that book, but you could have reminded him.

    c. Don would never have thought of that book, but you could of have reminded him.

    d. Don would never of thought of that book, but you could of reminded him.

2. Choose the correct sentence.

   a. The boy and girl are related.

   b. The boy and girl is related.

   c. The boy and girl was related.

   d. None of the above.

3. Choose the sentence with the correct grammar.

   a. There was scarcely no food in the pantry, because nobody ate at home.

   b. There was scarcely any food in the pantry, because nobody ate at home.

   c. There was scarcely any food in the pantry, because not nobody ate at home.

   d. There was scarcely no food in the pantry, because not nobody ate at home.

4. Choose the sentence with the correct grammar.

   a. Its important for you to know its official name; its called the Confederate Museum.

   b. It's important for you to know it's official name; it's called the Confederate Museum.

   c. It's important for you to know its official name; it's called the Confederate Museum.

   d. Its important for you to know it's official name; it's called the Confederate Museum.

5. Choose the sentence with the correct grammar.

   a. The man as well as his son has arrived.

   b. The man as well as his son have arrived.

   c. Both of the above.

   d. None of the above.

6. Thomas Edison _____ since he invented the light bulb, television, motion pictures, and phonograph.

    a. has always been known as the greatest inventor

    b. was always been known as the greatest inventor

    c. must have had been always known as the greatest inventor

    d. will had been known as the greatest inventor

7. The weatherman on Channel 6 said that this has been the

    a. most hottest summer on record

    b. most hotter summer on record

    c. hottest summer on record

    d. hotter summer on record

8. Although Joe is tall for his age, his brother Elliot is _____ of the two.

    a. the tallest

    b. more tallest

    c. the tall

    d. the taller

9. When KISS came to town, all of the tickets _____ before I could buy one.

    a. will be sold out

    b. had been sold out

    c. were being sold out

    d. was sold out

10. The rules of most sports _____ more complicated than we often realize.

    a. are

    b. is

    c. was

    d. has been

11. _____ won first place in the Western Division?

    a. Who

    b. Whom

    c. Which

    d. What

12. There are now several ways to listen to music, including radio, CDs, and Mp3 files _____ you can download onto an MP3 player.

    a. on which

    b. who

    c. whom

    d. which

13. Choose the sentence with the correct grammar.

    a. Each of them have to be given a ticket.

    b. Each of them is to be given a ticket.

    c. Each of them are to be given a ticket.

    d. None of the above.

14. Choose the correct spelling.

    a. maintainance

    b. maintenace

    c. maintanance

    d. maintenance

15. Choose the correct spelling.

    a. humoros

    b. humouros

    c. humorous

    d. humorus

16. Choose the correct spelling.

    a. mathematics

    b. mathmatics

    c. matematics

    d. mathamatics

17. Choose the sentence below with the correct punctuation.

    a. Ted and Janice, who had been friends for years, went on vacation together every summer.

    b. Ted and Janice, who had been friends for years, went on vacation together, every summer.

    c. Ted, and Janice who had been friends for years, went on vacation together every summer.

    d. Ted and Janice who had been friends for years went on vacation together every summer.

18. Choose the sentence with the correct capitalization.

a. The Sahara Desert is found in the northern part of Africa.

b. The Sahara Desert is found in the Northern part of Africa.

c. The Sahara desert is found in the northern part of Africa.

d. The Sahara desert is found in the Northern part of Africa.

19. She went with him to the dance.

What is the subject of this sentence?

a. She

b. Dance

c. Him

d. With

20. She studied long and hard and her marks showed it.

What is the predicate of this sentence?

a. Studied long and hard

b. Marks showed it

c. Showed it

d. None of the above

21. What is on the test?

What type of sentence is this?

a. Imperative

b. Interrogative

c. Exclamatory

d. Declarative

22. The aquarium featured brightly-colored tropical fish that came from the tropics.

What part of this sentence is redundant?

> a. Brightly-colored
> b. Tropical fish
> c. That came from the tropics
> d. Aquarium

23. Choose the correct sentence.

> a. Historians have been guessing the doctor was a woman for more than 100 years.
>
> b. Historians have been guessing for more than 100 years the doctor was a woman.
>
> c. Historians guessed the doctor was a woman for more than 100 years.
>
> d. None of the above.

24. Choose the correct sentence.

> a. None of us want to go to the party not even, if there will be live music.
>
> b. None of us want to go to the party, not even if there will be live music.
>
> c. None of us want to go to the party not even if there will be live music.
>
> d. None of us want to go to the party; not even if there will be live music.

25. Choose the correct sentence.

a. I own two dogs, a cat named Jeffrey, and Henry, the goldfish.

b. I own two dogs a cat, named Jeffrey, and Henry, the goldfish.

c. I own two dogs, a cat named Jeffrey; and Henry, the goldfish.

d. I own two dogs, a cat, named Jeffrey and Henry, the goldfish.

26. Choose the correct sentence.

a. During the years he was President, the country fought two wars.

b. During the years he was president, the country fought two wars.

c. During the years he was president, the Country fought two wars.

d. During the years he was President, the Country fought two wars.

27. Alice <u>jumped</u> when she saw the rabbit.

What part of speech is the underlined word?

a. Noun

b. Verb

c. Adjective

d. Adverb

28. Which of the following sentences contains a redundant phrase?

    a. I will be leaving shortly.

    b. I think the situation calls for a direct confrontation.

    c. The fish swam upstream with great difficulty.

    d. None of the above.

Directions: For each of the questions below, choose the word with the meaning best suited to the sentence based on the context.

29. Paul's rose bushes were being destroyed by Japanese beetles, so he invested in a good _____.

    a. Fungicide

    b. Fertilizer

    c. Sprinkler

    d. Pesticide

30. Because of a pituitary dysfunction, Karl lacked the necessary _____ to grow as tall as his father.

    a. Glands

    b. Hormones

    c. Vitamins

    d. Testosterone

Section III – Science

1. Describe the differences between genotypes and phenotypes.

    a. Phenotype refers to observed properties of an organism and genotype refers to the genes of an organism.

    b. Genotype refers to observed properties of an organism and phenotype refers to the genes of an organism.

    c. Phenotype refers to the DNA of an organism and genotype refers to the genes of an organism.

    d. Genotype refers to the DNA of an organism and phenotype refers to the genes of an organism.

2. A solution with a pH value of greater than 7 is

    a. Base.

    b. Acid.

    c. Neutral.

    d. None of the above.

3. Which statement below regarding Eukaryotic and prokaryotic cells is correct?

    a. Both are organelles

    b. Eukaryotic are not organelles

    c. Both have DNA

    d. Both have single membrane compartments

4. When we say that important traits for scientific classification are homologous, "homologous" means

a. Being shared among two or more animals with the same parent.

b. Being coincidentally shared by two totally different creatures.

c. Being inherited by the organisms' common ancestors.

d. Mutating beyond all reasonable expectations.

5. The manner in which instructions for building proteins, the basic structural molecules of living material are written in the DNA, is

a. Genotypic assignment.

b. Chromosome pattern.

c. Genetic code.

d. Genetic fingerprinting.

6. A _____ is a unit of inherited material, encoded by a strand of DNA and transcribed by RNA.

a. Allele

b. Phenotype

c. Gene

d. Genotype

7. Which, if any, of the following statements about meiosis are correct?

a. During meiosis, the number of chromosomes in the cell are halved.

b. Meiosis only occurs in eukaryotic cells.

c. Meiosis is the part of the life cycle that involves sexual reproduction.

d. All of these statements are correct.

8. A population of wolves expanded exponentially after a hunting ban. Within a few generations, their habitat exceeded its _____ _____.

    a. Carrying capacity

    b. Food source

    c. Population limit

    d. Supply capability

9. When a pouch in the large intestine becomes inflamed, this becomes an affliction known as

    a. Diverticulosis.

    b. Diverticulitis.

    c. Acid Reflux.

    d. Colon Cancer.

10. Why is detection of pathogens complicated?

    a. They evolve so quickly

    b. They die so quickly

    c. They are invisible

    d. They multiply so quickly

11. Photosynthesis is

    a. The process by which plants generate oxygen from carbon dioxide.

    b. The process by which plants generate carbon dioxide from oxygen.

    c. The process by which plants generate carbon dioxide and oxygen.

    d. None of the above.

12. Which, if any, of the following statements are false?

a. A mutation is a permanent change in the DNA sequence of a gene.

b. Mutations in a gene's DNA sequence can alter the amino acid sequence of the protein encoded by the gene.

c. Mutations in DNA sequences usually occur spontaneously.

d. Mutations in DNA sequences is caused by exposure to environmental agents such as sunshine.

13. Starting with the weakest, arrange the fundamental forces of nature in order of strength.

a. Gravity, Weak Nuclear Force, Electromagnetic Force, Strong Nuclear Force

b. Weak Nuclear Force, Gravity, Electromagnetic Force, Strong Nuclear Force

c. Strong Nuclear Force, Weak Nuclear Force, Electromagnetic Force, Gravity

d. Gravity, Strong Nuclear Force, Weak Nuclear Force, Electromagnetic Force

14. _____, which refers to the repeatability of measurement, does not require knowledge of the correct or true value.

a. Precision

b. Value

c. Certainty

d. Accuracy

15. Artificial selection

a. Is a process where desirable traits are systematically bred.

b. Is a process where traits become more or less common in a population.

c. Is a process where behaviors are favored.

d. None of the above.

16. Which of the following are not examples of vaporization?

a. Boiling

b. Evaporation

c. Condensation

d. All of the above

17. Describe the periodic table.

a. The periodic table is a tabular display of the chemical compounds organized on the basis of their atomic numbers, electron configurations, and recurring chemical properties.

b. The periodic table is a tabular display of the chemical elements, organized on the basis of their atomic numbers, electron configurations, and recurring chemical properties.

c. The periodic table is a tabular display of the chemical subatomic particles, organized on the basis of their atomic numbers, electron configurations, and recurring chemical properties.

d. None of the above.

**18. In terms of the scientific method, the term
_____ refers to the act of noticing or perceiving
something and/or recording a fact or occurrence.**

   a. Observation

   b. Diligence

   c. Perception

   d. Control

19. What is the difference, of any, between kinetic energy and potential energy?

   a. Kinetic energy is the energy of a body resulting from heat while potential energy is the energy possessed by an object that is chilled.

   b. Kinetic energy is the energy of a body resulting from motion while potential energy is the energy possessed by an object by virtue of its position or state, e.g., as in a compressed spring.

   c. There is no difference between kinetic and potential energy; all energy is the same.

   d. Potential energy is the energy of a body resulting from motion while kinetic energy is the energy possessed by an object by virtue of its position or state, e.g., as in a compressed spring.

20. What is the sequence of developmental stages through which members of a given species must pass?

   a. Life cycle

   b. Life expectancy

   c. Life sequence

   d. None of the above

21. Which one of the following best describes the function of a cell membrane?

   a. It controls the substances entering and leaving the

cell.

b. It keeps the cell in shape.

c. It controls the substances entering the cell.

d. It supports the cell structures.

22. Which of these is not a rank within the area of classification or taxonomy?

   a. Species

   b. Family

   c. Genus

   d. Relative position

23. A _____ is a statistic used as a measure of the dispersion or variation in a distribution.

   a. Normal distribution

   b. Range

   c. Outlier

   d. Standard deviation

24. Substances that deactivate catalysts are called

   a. Inhibitors.

   b. Catalytic poisons.

   c. Positive catalysts.

   d. None of the above.

25. Describe kinetic energy.

   a. Kinetic energy is the energy an object possesses due to its mass.

   b. Kinetic energy is the energy an object possesses due to its motion.

   c. Kinetic energy is the energy an object possesses due to its chemical properties.

   d. Kinetic energy is the stored energy an object possesses.

26. The interval of confidence around the measured value, such that the measured value is certain not to lie outside this stated interval, refers to the _____ of that value.

  a. Accuracy

  b. Error

  c. Uncertainty

  d. Measurement

27. What are the differences, if any, between arteries, veins, and capillaries?

  a. Veins carry oxygenated blood away from the heart, arteries return oxygen-depleted blood to the heart, and capillaries are thin-walled blood vessels in which gas/ nutrient/ waste exchange occurs.

  b. Capillaries carry oxygenated blood away from the heart, veins return oxygen-depleted blood to the heart, and capillaries are thin-walled blood vessels in which gas/ nutrient/ waste exchange occurs.

  c. There are no differences; all perform the same function in different parts of the body.

  d. Arteries carry oxygenated blood away from the heart, veins return oxygen-depleted blood to the heart, and capillaries are thin-walled blood vessels in which gas/ nutrient/ waste exchange occurs.

28. What part of the body starts inhalation?

  a. The lungs

  b. The diaphragm

  c. The larynx

  d. The kidneys

29. Another term for biological classification is:

　a.　Darwinian classification.

　b.　Animal classification.

　c.　Molecular classification.

　d.　Scientific classification.

30. What type of gene is not expressed as a trait unless inherited by both parents?

　a. Principal gene

　b. Latent gene

　c. Recessive gene

　d. Dominant gene

31. A _____ _____ is an approximation or simulation of a real system that omits all but the most essential variables of the system.

　a. Scientific method

　b. Independent variable

　c. Control group

　d. Scientific model

32. Neutrons are necessary within an atomic nucleus because

　a. They bind with protons via nuclear force.

　b. They bind with nuclei via nuclear force.

　c. They bind with protons via electromagnetic force.

　d. They bind with nuclei via electromagnetic force.

33. Which of the following statements is false?

    a. Most enzymes are proteins

    b. Enzymes are catalysts

    c. Most enzymes are inorganic

    d. Enzymes are large biological molecules

34. _____ are compounds that contain hydrogen, can dissolve in water to release hydrogen ions into solution, and, in an aqueous solution, can conduct electricity.

    a. Caustics

    b. Bases

    c. Acids

    d. Salts

35. What are the basic structural units of nucleic acids (DNA or RNA) whose sequence determines individual hereditary characteristics?

    a. Gene

    b. Nucleotide

    c. Phosphate

    d. Nitrogen base

36. List the classifications of organisms in order of size.

    a. Genus, Kingdom, Phylum/division, Class, Order, and Family Species

    b. Order, Kingdom, Phylum/division, Genus, Class, and Family Species

    c. Genus, Kingdom, Phylum/division, Class, Order, and Family Species

    d. Kingdom ,Genus, Phylum/division, Class, Order, and Family Species

    e. Family species, Order, Class, Phylum/division, Kingdom, and Genus

37. Where does digestion begin?

 a. In the throat

 b. In the stomach

 c. In the intestines

 d. In the mouth

38. What are the main components of the circulatory system?

 a. The heart, veins and blood vessels

 b. The heart, brain, and ears

 c. The nose, throat and ears

 d. The lungs, stomach, and kidneys

39. What is an example of a pathogen that the immune system detects?

 a. An atom

 b. A molecule

 c. A vitamin

 d. A virus

40. Explain chemical bonds.

 a. Chemical bonds are attractions between atoms that form chemical substances containing two or more atoms.

 b. Chemical bonds are attractions between protons that form chemical elements containing two or more atoms.

 c. Chemical bonds are two or more atoms that form chemical substances.

 d. None of the above.

41. Which of these is not an example of a function of the stomach in digestion?

    a. Storing food

    b. Cleansing food of impurities

    c. Mixing food with digestive juices

    d. Transferring food into the intestines

42. The exchange of oxygen for carbon dioxide takes place in the alveolar area of

    a. The throat.

    b. The ears.

    c. The appendix.

    d. The lungs.

43. The number of protons in the nucleus of an atom is the

    a. Atomic mass.

    b. Atomic weight.

    c. Atomic number.

    d. None of the above.

44. Natural selection is

    a. A process where biological traits become more common in a population.

    b. A process where biological traits become less common in a population.

    c. A process where biological traits become more or less common in a population.

    d. None of the above.

45. Sex chromosomes are designated as being "X" or "Y" chromosomes. In terms of sex chromosomes, what differences exist between males and females?

a. Females have two X chromosomes and males have one X chromosome and one Y chromosome.

b. Females have one X chromosome, and males have one X chromosome and one Y chromosome.

c. Females have one Y chromosome, while males have one X chromosome.

d. Females have one X chromosome and one Y chromosome, and males have two X chromosomes.

46. How does the immune system fight off disease?

a. By identifying and killing tumor cells and pathogens.

b. By creating new blood cells that fight disease.

c. By expelling infection through the blood stream.

d. By giving you energy to resist disease infections.

47. Identify the chemical properties of water.

a. Water has two hydrogen atoms covalently bonded to one oxygen atom.

b. Water has two oxygen atoms covalently bonded to one hydrogen atom.

c. Water has two hydrogen atoms polar covalently bonded to one oxygen atom.

d. Water has two oxygen atoms polar covalently bonded to one hydrogen atom.

48. Which of the following is not true of atomic theory?

a. Originated in the early 19th century with the work of John Dalton.

b. Is the field of physics that describes the characteristics and properties of atoms that make up matter.

c. Explains temperature as the momentum of atoms.

d. Explains macroscopic phenomena through the behavior of microscopic atoms.

Practice Test 1 - Quick Reference Answer Key

Section 1 – Reading

1. A
2. B
3. A
4. B
5. D
6. B
7. C
8. A
9. B
10. A
11. A
12. A
13. C
14. B
15. A
16. C
17. C
18. C
19. D
20. C
21. C
22. C
23. B
24. D
25. B
26. B
27. C
28. A
29. D
30. B
31. C
32. A
33. C
34. D

35. A

Section II – Math

1. A
2. D
3. D
4. B
5. C
6. C
7. A
8. A
9. B
10. A
11. B
12. D
13. B
14. A
15. C
16. B
17. A
18. B
19. C
20. C
21. D
22. C
23. D
24. D
25. B
26. B
27. B
28. B
29. A
30. D

Section III English

1. A
2. A

3. B
4. C
5. A
6. A
7. C
8. D
9. B
10. A
11. A
12. D
13. B
14. D
15. C
16. A
17. A
18. A
19. A
20. A
21. B
22. C
23. B
24. B
25. A
26. B
27. B
28. B
29. D
30. B

Section IV – Science

1. A
2. A
3. A
4. C
5. C
6. C
7. D
8. A
9. B
10. A

11. A
12. C
13. A
14. A
15. A
16. C
17. B
18. A
19. B
20. A
21. A
22. D
23. D
24. B
25. B
26. C
27. D
28. B
29. D
30. C
31. D
32. A
33. C
34. C
35. A
36. A
37. D
38. A
39. D
40. A
41. B
42. D
43. C
44. C
45. A
46. A
47. A
48. C

Answer Key with Explanations

Section 1 – Reading

1. A
Helen's parents hired Anne to teach Helen to communicate. Choice B is incorrect because the passage states Anne had trouble finding her way around, which means she could walk. Choice C is incorrect because you don't hire a teacher to teach someone to play. Choice D is incorrect because by age 6, if Helen had never eaten, she would have starved to death.

2. B
The correct answer because that fact is stated directly in the passage. The passage explains that Anne taught Helen to hear by allowing her to feel the vibrations in her throat.

3. A
We can infer that Anne is a patient teacher because she did not leave or lose her temper when Helen bit or hit her; she just kept trying to teach Helen. Choice B is incorrect because Anne taught Helen to read and talk. Choice C is incorrect because Anne could hear. She was partially blind, not deaf. Choice D is incorrect because it does not have to do with patience.

4. B
The passage states that it was hard for anyone but Anne to understand Helen when she spoke. Choice A is incorrect because the passage does not mention Helen spoke a foreign language. Choice C is incorrect because there is no mention of how quiet or loud Helen's voice was. Choice D is incorrect because we know from reading the passage that Helen did learn to speak.

5. D
This question tests the reader's summarization skills. The

question is asking very generally about the message of the passage, and the title, "Ways Characters Communicate in Theater," is one indication of that. The other choices A, B, and C are all directly from the text, and therefore readers may be inclined to select one of them, but are too specific to encapsulate the entirety of the passage and its message.

6. B

The paragraph on soliloquies mentions "To be or not to be," and it is from the context of that paragraph that readers may understand that because "To be or not to be" is a soliloquy, Hamlet will be introspective, or thoughtful, while delivering it. It is true that actors deliver soliloquies alone, and may be "solitary" (choice A), but "thoughtful" (choice B) is more true to the overall idea of the paragraph. Readers may choose C because drama and theater can be used interchangeably and the passage mentions that soliloquies are unique to theater (and therefore drama), but this answer is not specific enough to the paragraph in question. Readers may pick up on the theme of life and death and Hamlet's true intentions and select that he is "hopeless" (choice D), but those themes are not discussed either by this paragraph or passage, as a close textual reading and analysis confirms.

7. C

This question tests the reader's grammatical skills. Choice B seems logical, but parenthesis are actually considered to be a stronger break in a sentence than commas are, and along this line of thinking, actually disrupt the sentence more.

Choices A and D make comparisons between theater and film that are simply not made in the passage, and may or may not be true. This detail does clarify the statement that asides are most unique to theater by adding that it is not completely unique to theater, which may have been why the author didn't chose not to delete it and instead used parentheses to designate the detail's importance (choice C).

8. A

Low blood sugar occurs both in diabetics and healthy adults.

9. B

None of the statements are the author's opinion.

10. A

The author's purpose is the inform.

11. A

The only statement that is not a detail is, "A doctor can diagnosis this medical condition by asking the patient questions and testing."

12. A

This sentence is a recommendation.

13. C

Tips for a good night's sleep is the best alternative title for this article.

14. B

Mental activity is helpful for a good night's sleep is can not be inferred from this article.

15. A

From the passage, one disadvantage of taking naps is they may keep you awake at night.

16. C

Based on the partial table of contents, you would find information about natural selection in the ecology section on page 110.

17. C

To be infamous means to be remembered for an evil or terrible action. Therefore, the word infamy means to remember a bad or terrible thing. Choice A is incorrect because being famous is not the same as being infamous. Choice B is incorrect because the attack on Pearl Harbor was not good. Choice D is incorrect because Pearl Harbor was not forgotten.

18. C

Each other answer set contains the name of at least one country that was not part of the AXIS powers.

19. D

It is stated in the passage. Choice A is not correct because

there was no indication that Japan would attack San Diego
Choice B is incorrect because the attack on Pearl Harbor
was a surprise. Choice C is incorrect because Roosevelt was
not planning to attack Japan.

20. C

The passage clearly states that Japan planned a surprise
attack. They chose that early time to catch the U.S. military
off guard. Choice A is incorrect because the military does
not sleep late. Choice B is incorrect because there is no law
against bombing countries. Choice D is incorrect because it
makes no sense.

21. C

This question tests the reader's vocabulary skills. The uses
of the negatives "but" and "less," especially right next to each
other, may confuse readers into answering with choices A or
D, which list words that are antonyms to "militant." Readers
may also be confused by the comparison of healthy people
with what is being described as an overly healthy person--
both people are good, but the reader may look for which one
is "worse" in the comparison, and therefore stray toward
the antonym words. One key to understanding the meaning of "militant" if the reader is unfamiliar with it is to look
at the root of the word; readers can then easily associate
it with "military" and gain a sense of what the word signi-
fies: defence (especially considered that the immune system
defends the body). Choice C is correct over choice B because
"militant" is an adjective, just as the words in choice C are,
whereas the words in choice B are nouns.

22. C

This question tests the reader's understanding of function
within writing. The other choices are details included sur-
rounding the quoted text, and may therefore confuse the
reader. Choice A somewhat contradicts what is said earlier
in the paragraph, which is that tests and treatments are improving, and probably doctors are along with them, but the
paragraph doesn't actually mention doctors, and the subject
of the question is the medicine. Choice B may seem correct
to readers who aren't careful to understand that, while the
author does mention the large number of people affected,
the author is touching on the realities of living with allergies

rather about the likelihood of curing all allergies. Similarly, while the author does mention the "balance" of the body, which is easily associated with "wholesome," the author is not really making an argument and especially is not making an extreme statement that allergy medicines should be outlawed. Again, because the article's tone is on living with allergies, choice C is an appropriate choice that fits with the title and content of the text.

23. B
This question tests the reader's inference skills. The text does not state who is doing the recommending, but the use of the "patients," as well as the general context of the passage, lends itself to the logical partner, "doctors," choice B. The author does mention the recommendation but doesn't present it as her own (i.e. "I recommend that"), so choice A may be eliminated. It may seem plausible that people with allergies (choice D) may recommend medicines or products to other people with allergies, but the text does not necessarily support this interaction taking place. Choice C may be selected because the EpiPen is specifically mentioned, but the use of the phrase "such as" when it is introduced is not limiting enough to assume the recommendation is coming from its creators.

24. D
This question tests the reader's global understanding of the text. Choice D includes the main topics of the three body paragraphs, and isn't too focused on a specific aspect or quote from the text, as the other questions are, giving a skewed summary of what the author intended. The reader may be drawn to choice B because of the title of the passage and the use of words like "better," but the message of the passage is larger and more general than this.

25. B
Reading the document posted to the Human Resources website is optional.

26. B
The document is recommended changes and have not be implemented yet.

27. C

This question tests the reader's summarization skills. The use of the word "actually" in describing what kind of people poets are, as well as other moments like this, may lead readers to selecting choices B or D, but the author is more information than trying to persuade readers. The author gives no indication that she loves poetry (choice B) or that people, students specifically (D), should write poems. Choice A is incorrect because the style and content of this paragraph do not match those of a foreword; forewords usually focus on the history or ideas of a specific poem to introduce it more fully and help it stand out against other poems. The author here focuses on several poems and gives broad statements. Instead, she tells a kind of story about poems, giving three very broad time periods in which to discuss them, thereby giving a brief history of poetry, as choice C states.

28. A

This question tests the reader's summarization skills. Key words in the topic sentences of each of the paragraphs ("oldest," "Renaissance," "modern") should give the reader an idea that the author is moving chronologically. The opening and closing sentence-paragraphs are broad and talk generally. B seems reasonable, but epic poems are mentioned in two paragraphs, eliminating the idea that only new types of poems are used in each paragraph. Choice C is also easily eliminated because the author clearly mentions several different poets, groups of people, and poems. Choice D also seems reasonable, considering that the author does move from older forms of poetry to newer forms, but use of "so (that)" makes this statement false, for the author gives no indication that she is rushing (the paragraphs are about the same size) or that she prefers modern poetry.

29. D

This question tests the reader's attention to detail. The key word is "invented"-- it ties together the Mesopotamians, who invented the written word, and the fact that they, as the inventors, also invented and used poetry. The other selections focus on other details mentioned in the passage, such as that the Renaissance's admiration of the Greeks (choice C) and that Beowulf is in Old English (choice A). Choice B may seem like an attractive answer because it is unlike the others and because the idea of heroes seems rooted in ancient and early civilizations.

30. B
This question tests the reader's vocabulary and contextual-ization skills. "Telling" is not an unusual word, but it may be used here in a way that is not familiar to readers, as an adjective rather than a verb in gerund form. A may seem like the obvious answer to a reader looking for a verb to match the use they are familiar with. If the reader understands that the word is being used as an adjective and that choice A is a ploy, they may opt to select choice D, "wordy," but it does not make sense in context. Choice C can be easily eliminat-ed, and doesn't have any connection to the paragraph or passage. "Significant" (choice B) makes sense contextually, especially relative to the phrase "give insight" used later in the sentence.

31. C
Wind is the highest source of renewable energy in Scotland. The other choices are either not mentioned at all or not men-tioned in the context for how fast they are growing.

32. A
Most Scottish citizens agree with the Government's plan due to the concern for current and future needs.

Choice B is a good choice but not why the majority agree. Choice C is meant to mislead the as they are clearly in sight. Choice D is a good 'common sense' choice but mentioned specifically in the text.

33. C
The up-front cost is expensive.
The other choices may appear to be correct, and even be common sense, but they are not specifically mentioned in the paragraph.

34. D
The best way to describe the paragraphs description of wind energy is clean and renewable but fluctuating.
The other choices are good descriptions of wind energy, but not the best way to describe the article.

35. A
The Save the Children's fund has raised $12,000 out of $20,000, or 12/20. Simplifying, 12/20 = 3/5

Section II – Math

1. A
1/3 X 3/4 = 3/12 = 1/4
To multiply fractions, multiply the numerator and denominator.

2. D
The question asks for approximate cost, so work with round numbers. The jacket costs $545.00 so we can round up to $550. 10% of $550 is 55. We can round down to $50, which is easier to work with. $550 - $50 is $500. The jacket will cost about $500.

The actual cost will be 10% X 545 = $54.50
545 – 54.50 = $490.50

3. D
3.14 + 2.73 = 5.87 and 5.87 + 23.7 = 29.57

4. B
Spent 15%, so 100% - 15% = 85%

5. C
To convert a decimal to a fraction, take the places of decimal as your denominator, here, 2, so in 0.27, '7' is in the 100th place, so the fraction is 27/100 and 0.33 becomes 33/100.

Next estimate the answer quickly to eliminate obvious wrong choices. 27/100 is about 1/4 and 33/100 is 1/3. 1/3 is slightly larger than 1/4, and 1/4 + 1/4 is 1/2, so the answer will be slightly larger than 1/2.
Looking at the choices, Choice A can be eliminated since 3/6 = 1/2. Choice D, 2/7 is less than 1/2 and be eliminated. The answer is going to be Choice B or Choice C.

Do the calculation, 0.27 + 0.33 = 0.60 and 0.60 = 60/100 = 3/5, Choice C is correct.

6. C
This is an easy question, and shows how you can solve some questions without doing the calculations. The question is, 8 is what percent of 40. Take easy percentages for an approximate answer and see what you get.

10% is easy to calculate because you can drop the zero, or move the decimal point. 10% of 40 = 4, and 8 = 2 X 4, so, 8 must be 2 X 10% = 20%.

Here are the calculations which confirm the quick approximation.
8/40 = X/100 = 8 * 100 / 40X = 800/40 = X = 20

7. A
According to the graph, oil consumption peaked in 2011.

8. A
2 + a number divided by 7.
(2 + X) divided by 7.
(2 + X)/7

9. B
.4/100 * 36 = .4 * 36/100 = .144

10. A
5 mg/10/mg X 1 tab/1 = .5 tablets

11. B
Step 1: Set up the formula to calculate the dose to be given in mg as per weight of the child:- Dose ordered X Weight in Kg – Dose to be given
Step 2: 20 mg X 12 kg = 240 mg
240 mg/80 mg X 1 tab/1 = 240/80 = 3 tablets

12. D
Indonesia is growing the fastest at about 30%.

13. B
$(4)(3)^3 = (4)(27) = 108$

14. A
MCMXC is 1990. 1000 + (1000 – 100) + (100 – 10) = 1990

15. C
4 quarts = 1 gallon, 16 quarts = 16/4 = 4 gallons. Conversion problems are easy to get confused. One way to think of them is which is larger - quarts or gallons? Gallons are larger, so if you are converting from quarts to gallons the number of gallons will be a smaller number. Keeping that in mind, you can do a 'common-sense' check your answer.

16. B
0.45 kg = 1 pound, 1 kg. = 1/0.45 and 45 kg = 1/0.45 x 45 = 99.208, or 100 pounds.

17. A
Three plus a number times 7 equals 42. Let X be the number.
(3 + X) times 7 = 42
7(3 + X) = 42

18. B
Number of absent students = 83 – 72 = 11

Percentage of absent students is found by proportioning the number of absent students to total number of students in the class = 11 * 100/83 = 13.25

Checking the answers, we round 13.25 to the nearest whole number: 13%

19. C
To solve for x, first simplify the equation
5x + 2x + 14 = 14x – 7
7x - 14x = -14 -7
-7x = -21
x = -21/-7
x = 3

20. C
5z + 5 = 3z + 6 + 11
5z -3z + 5 = 6 + 11
5z – 3z = 6 + 11 -5
2z = 17 – 5

$2z = 12$

$z = 12/2$

$z = 6$

21. D

Price increased by $5 ($25-$20). To calculate the percent increase:

$5/20 = X/100$

$500 = 20X$

$X = 500/20$

$X = 25\%$

22. C

The ratio is 2 to 8, or 1:4.

23. D

2 glasses are broken for 43 customers so 1 glass breaks for every 43/2 customers served, therefore 10 glasses implies $(43/2) \cdot 10 = 215$ customers.

24. D

As the lawn is square , the length of one side will be the square root of the area. $\sqrt{62,500} = 250$ meters. So, the perimeter is found by 4 times the length of the side of the square:

$250 \cdot 4 = 1000$ meters.

Since each meter costs $5.5, the total cost of the fence will be $1000 \cdot 5.5 = \$5,500$.

25. B

$5n + (19 - 2) = 67$, $5n + 17 = 67$, $5n = 67 - 17$, $5n = 50$, $n = 50/5 = 10$

26. B

Day	Absent	Present	%
Monday	5	40	88.88%
Tuesday	9	36	80.00%
Wednesday	4	41	91.11%
Thursday	10	35	77.77%
Friday	6	39	86.66%

Sum of the percent attendance is 424.42. Divide by 5 for the average, 424.42/5 = 84.884. Round up to 85%.

27. B
The distribution is done in three different rates and amounts:

$6.4 per 20 kilograms to 15 shops ... 20•15 = 300 kilograms distributed

$3.4 per 10 kilograms to 12 shops ... 10•12 = 120 kilograms distributed

550 - (300 + 120) = 550 - 420 = 130 kilograms left. This amount is distributed by 5 kilogram portions. So, this means that there are 130/5 = 26 shops.

$1.8 per 130 kilograms.

We need to find the amount he earned overall these distributions.

$6.4 per 20 kilograms : 6.4•15 = $96 for 300 kilograms

$3.4 per 10 kilograms : 3.4•12 = $40.8 for 120 kilograms

$1.8 per 5 kilograms : 1.8•26 = $46.8 for 130 kilograms

So, he earned 96 + 40.8 + 46.8 = $ 183.6

The total distribution cost is given as $10

The profit is found by: Money earned - money spent ... It is important to remember that he bought 550 kilograms of potatoes for $165 at the beginning:

Profit = 183.6 - 10 - 165 = $8.6

28. B
We check the fractions taking place in the question. We see that there is a "half" (that is 1/2) and 3/7. So, we multiply the denominators of these fractions to decide how to name the total money. We say that Mr. Johnson has 14x at the beginning; he gives half of this, meaning 7x, to his family. $250 to his landlord. He has 3/7 of his money left. 3/7 of

14x is equal to:

14x•(3/7) = 6x

So,

Spent money is: 7x + 250

Unspent money is: 6x

Total money is: 14x

We write an equation: total money = spent money + unspent money

14x = 7x + 250 + 6x

14x - 7x - 6x = 250

x = 250

We are asked to find the total money that is 14x:

14x = 14 * 250 = $3500

29. A
The probability that the 1st ball drawn is red = 4/11
The probability that the 2nd ball drawn is green = 5/10
The combined probability will then be 4/11 X 5/10 = 20/110 = 2/11

30. D
First calculate total square feet, which is 15 * 24 = 360 ft^2.
Next, convert this vaue to square yards, (1 yards^2 = 9 ft^2) which is 360/9 = 40 yards^2. At $0.50 per square yard, the total cost is 40 * 0.50 = $20.

Section III English

1. A
The third conditional is used for talking about an unreal situation (a situation that did not happen) in the past. For

example, "If I had studied harder, [if clause] I would have passed the exam" [main clause]. This has the same meaning as, "I failed the exam, because I didn't study hard enough."

2. A
Use a plural verb form for two subjects linked by "and."

3. B
In double negative sentences, one negative is replaced with "any."

4. C
"It's" is a contraction for it is or it has. "Its" is a possessive pronoun.

5. A
When two subjects are linked by "with" or "as well," use the verb form that matches the first subject.

6. A
The sentence requires the past perfect "has always been known." This is the only grammatically correct choice.

7. C
The superlative, "hottest," is used when expressing a temperature greater than that of anything to which it is being compared.

8. D
When comparing two items, use "the taller." When comparing more than two items, use "the tallest."

9. B
The past perfect form is used to describe an event that occurred in the past and prior to another event. Here there are two things that happened, both of them in the past, and something the person wanted to do.

Event 1: Kiss came to town
Event 2: All the tickets sold out
What I wanted to do: Buy a ticket

The events are arranged:

When KISS came to town, all the tickets **had been sold out** before I could buy one.

10. A
The subject is "rules" so the present tense plural form, "are," is used to agree with "realize."

11. A
"Who" is correct because the question uses an active construction. "To whom was first place given?" is a passive construction.

12. D
"Which" is correct, because the files are objects and not people.

13. B
Use a singular verb with either, each, neither, everyone and many.

14. D
Maintenance is the correct spelling.

15. C
Humorous is the correct spelling.

16. A
Mathematics is the correct spelling.

17. A
Use a comma to separate phrases.

18. A
The Sahara Desert is a proper name so capitalized. The names of countries, ie Africa are capitalized.

19. A
'She' is the simple subject of this sentence.

20. A
The simple predicate is 'studied long and hard.' The predicate of a sentence is the action performed by the subject.

21. B
This is an interrogative sentence.

22. C
It is not necessary to say the fish came from the topics, since we already know they are tropical.

23. B
The correct sentence is
Historians have been guessing for more than 100 years the doctor was a woman.

Here the phrase 'for more than 100 years' refers to how long historians have been guessing, and not to how long the doctor has been a woman.

24. B
Use a comma separates independent clauses. None of us wants to go to the party, not even if there will be live music.

25. A
This is an example where a comma appears before 'and,' but is disambiguating. Without the comma, the sentence would be "I own two dogs, a cat named Jeffrey and Henry, the goldfish." This means there is a cat named Jeffrey and Henry, and a goldfish with no name mentioned. The comma appears to show the distinction.

I own two dogs, a cat named Jeffrey, and Henry, the goldfish.

26. B
President is not capitalized unless used with a name as in, President Obama.

27. B
'Jumped' is a verb. Verbs describe an action, state, or occurrence.

28. B
A confrontation is a head-on conflict, so a direct confrontation is redundant.

29. D
Pesticide: NOUN a substance, usually synthetic although sometimes biological, used to kill or contain the activities of pests.

30. B
Hormones: NOUN any substance produced by one tissue and conveyed by the bloodstream to another to effect physiological activity.

Section IV – Science

1. A
Phenotype refers to observed properties of an organism and genotype refers to the genes of an organism.

2. A
A solution with a pH value of greater than 7 is base.

3. A
Eukaryotic and prokaryotic cells are both organelles.

4. C
Homologous is being inherited by the organisms' common ancestors. An example would be feathers and hair—both of which were structures that shared a common ancestral trait.

5. C
The manner in which instructions for building proteins, the basic structural molecules of living material are written in the DNA is a **genetic code**.

6. C
A gene is a unit of inherited material, encoded by a strand of DNA and transcribed by RNA.

7. D
All these statements are correct.

     a. During meiosis, the number of chromosomes in the cell are halved.

b. Meiosis only occurs in eukaryotic cells.

c. Meiosis is the part of the life cycle that involves sexual reproduction.

8. A Carrying capacity
An area's carrying capacity is the maximum number of animals of a given species that area can support during the harshest part of the year.

9. B
Diverticulitis is a pouch in the large intestine becomes inflamed.

10. A
Detection of pathogens can be complicated because they evolve so quickly.

11. A
Photosynthesis is the process by which plants and other photoautotrophs generate carbohydrates and oxygen from carbon dioxide, water, and light energy in chloroplasts.

12. C
Mutations in DNA sequences usually occur spontaneously is false.

13. A
Starting with the weakest, the fundamental forces of nature in order of strength are, Gravity, Weak nuclear force, Electromagnetic force, Strong nuclear force.

14. A
Precision, which refers to the repeatability of measurement, does not require knowledge of the correct or true value.

15. A
Artificial selection is a process where desirable traits are systematically bred.

16. C
Condensation is not an example of vaporization. Boiling and

evaporation are both examples of vaporization. Condensation is the process by which matter transitions from a gas into a liquid.

17. B
The periodic table is a tabular display of the chemical elements, organized by their atomic numbers, electron configurations, and recurring chemical properties.

18. A
In terms of the scientific method, the term observation refers to the act of noticing or perceiving something and/or recording a fact or occurrence.

19. B
Kinetic energy is the energy of a body that results from motion while potential energy is the energy possessed by an object by virtue of its position or state, e.g., as in a compressed spring.

20. A
A life cycle is the sequence of developmental stages through which members of a given species must pass.

21. A
The cell membrane is a biological membrane that separates the interior of all cells from the outside environment. The cell membrane is selectively permeable to ions and organic molecules and controls the movement of substances in and out of cells. [16]

22. D
Relative position. Ranks include Domain, Kingdom, Phylum, Class, Order, Family, Genus, and Species.

23. D
A Standard deviation is a statistic used as a measure of the dispersion or variation in a distribution.

24. B
Substances that deactivate catalysts are called catalytic

poisons.

25. B
Kinetic energy is the energy an object possesses due to its motion.

26. C
The interval of confidence around the measured value, such that the measured value is certain not to lie outside the stated interval refers to the **uncertainty** of that value.

27. D
Arteries carry oxygenated blood away from the heart, veins return oxygen-depleted blood to the heart, and capillaries are thin-walled blood vessels in which gas/ nutrient/ waste exchange occurs.

Note: An easy way to remember the difference between an artery and a vein is that Arteries carry Away from the heart.

28. B
The thoracic diaphragm, is a skeletal muscle across the bottom of the rib cage. The thoracic membrane is important in respiratory function.

29. D
Scientific classification. The two phrases are interchangeable, although the former seems to more accurately reflect the purpose of classification: to categorize biological units.

30. C
A recessive gene is not expressed as a trait unless inherited by both parents.

31. D
A scientific model is an approximation or simulation of a real system that omits all but the most essential variables of the system.

32. A
Neutrons are necessary within an atomic nucleus as they

bind with protons via the nuclear force.

33. C
The following statement is false - Most enzymes are inorganic.

34. C
Acids are compounds that contain hydrogen and can dissolve in water to release hydrogen ions into solution.

35. A
Genes determine individual hereditary characteristics.

36. A
The groups into which organisms are classified are called taxa and include, in order of size, Genus, Kingdom, Phylum/division, Class, Order, and Family Species.

37. D
Digestion begins in the mouth.

38. A
The main components of the circulatory system are the heart, veins and blood vessels.

39. D
An example of a pathogen that the immune system detects is a virus.

40. A
Chemical bonds are attractions between atoms that form chemical substances containing two or more atoms.

41. B
Cleansing food of impurities is not an example of a function of the stomach in digestion.

42. D
The exchange of oxygen for carbon dioxide takes place in the alveolar area of the lungs.

43. C

In chemistry, the number of protons in the nucleus of an atom is known as the atomic number, which determines the chemical element to which the atom belongs.

44. C

Natural selection is a process where biological traits become more or less common in a population.

45. A

Females have two X chromosomes and males have one X chromosome and one Y chromosome.

46. A

The immune system fight off disease by identifying and killing tumor cells and pathogens.

47. A

Water has two hydrogen atoms covalently bonded to one oxygen atom.

48. C

Choice C (Atomic theory explains temperature as the momentum of atoms.) is incorrect because atomic theory explains temperature as the motion of atoms (faster = hotter), not the momentum. The momentum of atoms explains the outward pressure that they exert.

Practice Test Questions Set 2

Section I – Reading

Questions: 35
Time: 35 Minutes

Section II – Math

Questions: 30
Time: 30 Minutes

Section III – English and Language Usage

Questions: 30
Time: 30 Minutes

Section IV – Science

Questions: 48
Time: 40 Minutes

The questions below are not the same as you will find on the TEAS® - that would be too easy! And nobody knows what the questions will be and they change all the time. Below are general questions that cover the same subject areas as the TEAS®. So, while the format and exact wording of the questions may differ slightly, and change from year to year, if you can answer the questions below, you will have no problem with the TEAS®.

For the best results, take these practice test questions as if it were the real exam. Set aside time when you will not be disturbed, and a location that is quiet and free of distractions. Read the instructions carefully, read each question carefully, and answer to the best of your ability.

You are given 209 minutes to complete the full TEAS® exam.

Use the bubble answer sheets provided. When you have completed the practice test questions, check your answer against the Answer Key and read the explanation provided.

Do not attempt more than one set of practice test questions in one day. After completing the first practice test, wait two or three days before attempting the second set of questions.

Section I – Reading Answer Sheet

	A	B	C	D	E		A	B	C	D	E
1	○	○	○	○	○	21	○	○	○	○	○
2	○	○	○	○	○	22	○	○	○	○	○
3	○	○	○	○	○	23	○	○	○	○	○
4	○	○	○	○	○	24	○	○	○	○	○
5	○	○	○	○	○	25	○	○	○	○	○
6	○	○	○	○	○	26	○	○	○	○	○
7	○	○	○	○	○	27	○	○	○	○	○
8	○	○	○	○	○	28	○	○	○	○	○
9	○	○	○	○	○	29	○	○	○	○	○
10	○	○	○	○	○	30	○	○	○	○	○
11	○	○	○	○	○	31	○	○	○	○	○
12	○	○	○	○	○	32	○	○	○	○	○
13	○	○	○	○	○	33	○	○	○	○	○
14	○	○	○	○	○	34	○	○	○	○	○
15	○	○	○	○	○	35	○	○	○	○	○
16	○	○	○	○	○						
17	○	○	○	○	○						
18	○	○	○	○	○						
19	○	○	○	○	○						
20	○	○	○	○	○						

Section II – Math – Answer Sheet

A B C D E   A B C D E

1 ◯◯◯◯◯   21 ◯◯◯◯◯
2 ◯◯◯◯◯   22 ◯◯◯◯◯
3 ◯◯◯◯◯   23 ◯◯◯◯◯
4 ◯◯◯◯◯   24 ◯◯◯◯◯
5 ◯◯◯◯◯   25 ◯◯◯◯◯
6 ◯◯◯◯◯   26 ◯◯◯◯◯
7 ◯◯◯◯◯   27 ◯◯◯◯◯
8 ◯◯◯◯◯   28 ◯◯◯◯◯
9 ◯◯◯◯◯   29 ◯◯◯◯◯
10 ◯◯◯◯◯   30 ◯◯◯◯◯
11 ◯◯◯◯◯
12 ◯◯◯◯◯
13 ◯◯◯◯◯
14 ◯◯◯◯◯
15 ◯◯◯◯◯
16 ◯◯◯◯◯
17 ◯◯◯◯◯
18 ◯◯◯◯◯
19 ◯◯◯◯◯
20 ◯◯◯◯◯

Section III – English and Language Usage Answer Sheet

	A	B	C	D	E		A	B	C	D	E
1	○	○	○	○	○	21	○	○	○	○	○
2	○	○	○	○	○	22	○	○	○	○	○
3	○	○	○	○	○	23	○	○	○	○	○
4	○	○	○	○	○	24	○	○	○	○	○
5	○	○	○	○	○	25	○	○	○	○	○
6	○	○	○	○	○	26	○	○	○	○	○
7	○	○	○	○	○	27	○	○	○	○	○
8	○	○	○	○	○	28	○	○	○	○	○
9	○	○	○	○	○	29	○	○	○	○	○
10	○	○	○	○	○	30	○	○	○	○	○
11	○	○	○	○	○						
12	○	○	○	○	○						
13	○	○	○	○	○						
14	○	○	○	○	○						
15	○	○	○	○	○						
16	○	○	○	○	○						
17	○	○	○	○	○						
18	○	○	○	○	○						
19	○	○	○	○	○						
20	○	○	○	○	○						

Section IV – Science Answer Sheet

	A	B	C	D	E		A	B	C	D	E
1	○	○	○	○	○	26	○	○	○	○	○
2	○	○	○	○	○	27	○	○	○	○	○
3	○	○	○	○	○	28	○	○	○	○	○
4	○	○	○	○	○	29	○	○	○	○	○
5	○	○	○	○	○	30	○	○	○	○	○
6	○	○	○	○	○	31	○	○	○	○	○
7	○	○	○	○	○	32	○	○	○	○	○
8	○	○	○	○	○	33	○	○	○	○	○
9	○	○	○	○	○	34	○	○	○	○	○
10	○	○	○	○	○	35	○	○	○	○	○
11	○	○	○	○	○	36	○	○	○	○	○
12	○	○	○	○	○	37	○	○	○	○	○
13	○	○	○	○	○	38	○	○	○	○	○
14	○	○	○	○	○	39	○	○	○	○	○
15	○	○	○	○	○	40	○	○	○	○	○
16	○	○	○	○	○	41	○	○	○	○	○
17	○	○	○	○	○	42	○	○	○	○	○
18	○	○	○	○	○	43	○	○	○	○	○
19	○	○	○	○	○	44	○	○	○	○	○
20	○	○	○	○	○	45	○	○	○	○	○
21	○	○	○	○	○	46	○	○	○	○	○
22	○	○	○	○	○	47	○	○	○	○	○
23	○	○	○	○	○	48	○	○	○	○	○
24	○	○	○	○	○	49	○	○	○	○	○
25	○	○	○	○	○	50	○	○	○	○	○

Section I - Reading

Questions 1 - 4 refer to the following passage.

Passage 1 - The Crusades

In 1095 Pope Urban II proclaimed the First Crusade with the intent and stated goal to restore Christian access to holy places in and around Jerusalem. Over the next 200 years there were 6 major crusades and numerous minor crusades in the fight for control of the "Holy Land." Historians are divided on the real purpose of the Crusades, some believing that it was part of a purely defensive war against Islamic conquest; some see them as part of a long-running conflict at the frontiers of Europe; and others see them as confident, aggressive, papal-led expansion attempts by Western Christendom. The impact of the crusades was profound, and judgment of the Crusaders ranges from laudatory to highly critical. However, all agree that the Crusades and wars waged during those crusades were brutal and often bloody. Several hundred thousand Roman Catholic Christians joined the Crusades, they were Christians from all over Europe.

Europe at the time was under the Feudal System, so while the Crusaders made vows to the Church they also were beholden to their Feudal Lords. This led to the Crusaders not only fighting the Saracen, the commonly used word for Muslim at the time, but also each other for power and economic gain in the Holy Land. This infighting between the Crusaders is why many historians hold the view that the Crusades were simply a front for Europe to invade the Holy Land for economic gain in the name of the Church. Another factor contributing to this theory is that while the army of crusaders marched towards Jerusalem they pillaged the land as they went. The church and feudal Lords vowing to return the land to its original beauty, and inhabitants, this rarely happened though as the Lords often kept the land for themselves. A full 800 years after the Crusades, Pope John Paul II expressed his sorrow for the massacre of innocent people and the lasting damage the Medieval church caused in that area of the World.

1. What is the tone of this article?

    a. Subjective

    b. Objective

    c. Persuasive

    d. None of the Above

2. What can all historians agree on concerning the Crusades?

    a. It achieved great things

    b. It stabilized the Holy Land

    c. It was bloody and brutal

    d. It helped defend Europe from the Byzantine Empire

3. What impact did the feudal system have on the Crusades

    a. It unified the Crusaders

    b. It helped gather volunteers

    c. It had no effect on the Crusades

    d. It led to infighting, causing more damage than good

4. What does Saracen mean?

    a. Muslim

    b. Christian

    c. Knight

    d. Holy Land

Questions 5-8 refer to the following passage.

ABC Electric Warranty

ABC Electric Company warrants that its products are free from defects in material and workmanship. Subject to the conditions and limitations set forth below, ABC Electric will, at its option, either repair or replace any part of its products that prove defective due to improper workmanship or materials.

This limited warranty does not cover any damage to the product from improper installation, accident, abuse, misuse, natural disaster, insufficient or excessive electrical supply, abnormal mechanical or environmental conditions, or any unauthorized disassembly, repair, or modification.

This limited warranty also does not apply to any product on which the original identification information has been altered, or removed, has not been handled or packaged correctly, or has been sold as second-hand.

This limited warranty covers only repair, replacement, refund or credit for defective ABC Electric products, as provided above.

5. I tried to repair my ABC Electric blender, but could not, so can I get it repaired under this warranty?

    a. Yes, the warranty still covers the blender

    b. No, the warranty does not cover the blender

    c. Uncertain. ABC Electric may or may not cover repairs under this warranty

6. My ABC Electric fan is not working. Will ABC Electric provide a new one or repair this one?

    a. ABC Electric will repair my fan

    b. ABC Electric will replace my fan

    c. ABC Electric could either replace or repair my fan can request either a replacement or a repair.

7. My stove was damaged in a flood. Does this warranty cover my stove?

    a. Yes, it is covered.

    b. No, it is not covered.

    c. It may or may not be covered.

    d. ABC Electric will decide if it is covered

8. Which of the following is an example of improper workmanship?

    a. Missing parts

    b. Defective parts

    c. Scratches on the front

    d. None of the above

Questions 9 – 12 refer to the following passage.

Passage 2 - Women and Advertising

Only in the last few generations have media messages been so widespread and so readily seen, heard, and read by so many people. Advertising is an important part of both selling and buying anything from soap to cereal to jeans. For whatever reason, more consumers are women than are men. Media message are subtle but powerful, and more attention has been paid lately to how these message affect women. Of all the products that women buy, makeup, clothes, and other stylistic or cosmetic products are among the most popular. This means that companies focus their advertising on women, promising them that their product will make her feel, look, or smell better than the next company's product will. This competition has resulted in advertising that is more and more ideal and less and less possible for everyday women. However, because women do look to these ideals and the products they represent as how they can potentially become, many women have developed unhealthy attitudes about themselves when they have failed to become those ideals.

In recent years, more companies have tried to change advertisements to be healthier for women. This includes featuring models of more sizes and addressing a huge outcry against unfair tools such as airbrushing and photo editing. There is debate about what the right balance between real and ideal is, because fashion is also considered art and some changes are made to purposefully elevate fashionable products and signify that they are creative, innovative, and the work of individual people. Artists want their freedom protected as much as women do, and advertising agencies are often caught in the middle.

Some claim that the companies who make these changes are not doing enough. Many people worry that there are still not enough models of different sizes and different ethnicities. Some people claim that companies use this healthier type of advertisement not for the good of women, but because they would like to sell products to the women who are looking for these kinds of messages. This is also a hard balance to find: companies do need to make money, and women do need to feel respected.

While the focus of this change has been on women, advertising can also affect men, and this change will hopefully be a lesson on media for all consumers.

9. The second paragraph states that advertising focuses on women

    a. to shape what the ideal should be

    b. because women buy makeup

    c. because women are easily persuaded

    d. because of the types of products that women buy

10. According to the passage, fashion artists and female consumers are at odds because

    a. there is a debate going on and disagreement drives people apart

    b. both of them are trying to protect their freedom to do something

    c. artists want to elevate their products above the reach of women

    d. women are creative, innovative, individual people

11. The author uses the phrase "for whatever reason" in this passage to

    a. keep the focus of the paragraph on media messages and not on the differences between men and women

    b. show that the reason for this is unimportant

    c. argue that it is stupid that more women are consumers than men

    d. show that he or she is tired of talking about why media messages are important

12. This passage suggests that

    a. advertising companies are still working on making their messages better

    b. all advertising companies seek to be more approachable for women

    c. women are only buying from companies that respect them

    d. artists could stop producing fashionable products if they feel bullied

Questions 13 - 16 refer to the following passage.

FDR, the Treaty of Versailles, and the Fourteen Points

At the conclusion of World War I, those who had won the war and those who were forced to admit defeat welcomed the end of the war and expected that a peace treaty would be signed. The American president, Franklin D. Roosevelt, played an important part in proposing what the agreements should be and did so through his Fourteen Points. World War I had begun in 1914 when an Austrian archduke was assassinated, leading to a domino effect that pulled the world's most powerful countries into war on a large scale. The war catalyzed the creation and use of deadly weapons that had not previously existed, resulting in a great loss of soldiers on both sides of the fighting. More than 9 million soldiers were killed.

The United States agreed to enter the war right before it ended, and many believed that its decision to become finally involved brought on the end of the war. FDR made it very clear that the U.S. was entering the war for moral reasons and had an agenda focused on world peace. The Fourteen Points were individual goals and ideas (focused on peace, free trade, open communication, and self reliance) that FDR wanted the power nations to strive for now that the war had concluded. He was optimistic and had many ideas about what could be accomplished through and during the post-war peace. However, FDR's fourteen points were poorly received when he presented them to the leaders of other world powers, many of whom wanted only to help their own countries and to punish the Germans for fueling the war, and they fell by the wayside. World War II was imminent, for Germany lost everything.

Some historians believe that the other leaders who participated in the Treaty of Versailles weren't receptive to the Fourteen Points because World War I was fought almost entirely on European soil, and the United States lost much less than did the other powers. FDR was in a unique position to determine the fate of the war, but doing it on his own terms did not help accomplish his goals. This is only one historical example of how the United State has tried to use its power as an important country, but found itself limited because of geological or ideological factors.

13. The main idea of this passage is that

    a. World War I was unfair because no fighting took place in America

    b. World War II happened because of the Treaty of Versailles

    c. the power the United States has to help other countries also prevents it from helping other countries

    d. Franklin D. Roosevelt was one of the United States' smartest presidents

14. According to the second paragraph, World War I started because

    a. an archduke was assassinated

    b. weapons that were more deadly had been developed

    c. a domino effect of allies agreeing to help each other

    d. the world's most powerful countries were large

15. The author includes the detail that 9 million soldiers were killed

    a. to demonstrate why European leaders were hesitant to accept peace

    b. to show the reader the dangers of deadly weapons

    c. to make the reader think about which countries lost the most soldiers

    d. to demonstrate why World War II was imminent

16. According to this passage, it can be understood that the word catalyzed means

    a. analyzed

    b. sped up

    c. invented

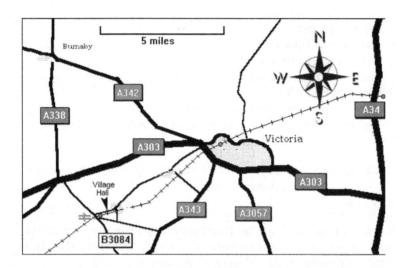

17. Approximately how far is Victoria to Burnaby?

    a. About 10 miles

    b. About 5 miles

    c. About 15 miles

    d. About 20 miles

18. How is the Village Hall from Victoria?

    a. About 10 miles

    b. About 5 miles

    c. About 15 miles

    d. About 20 miles

Questions 19 - 23 refer to the following passage.

Chocolate Chip Cookies

3/4 cup sugar
3/4 cup packed brown sugar
1 cup butter, softened
2 large eggs, beaten
1 teaspoon vanilla extract
2 1/4 cups all-purpose flour
1 teaspoon baking soda
3/4 teaspoon salt
2 cups semisweet chocolate chips
If desired, 1 cup chopped pecans, or chopped walnuts.
Preheat oven to 375 degrees.

Mix sugar, brown sugar, butter, vanilla and eggs in a large bowl. Stir in flour, baking soda, and salt. The dough will be very stiff.

Stir in chocolate chips by hand with a sturdy wooden spoon. Add the pecans, or other nuts, if desired. Stir until the chocolate chips and nuts are evenly dispersed.

Drop dough by rounded tablespoonfuls 2 inches apart onto a cookie sheet.

Bake 8 to 10 minutes or until light brown. Cookies may look underdone, but they will finish cooking after you take them out of the oven.

19. What is the correct order for adding these ingredients?

    a. Brown sugar, baking soda, chocolate chips

    b. Baking soda, brown sugar, chocolate chips

    c. Chocolate chips, baking soda, brown sugar

    d. Baking soda, chocolate chips, brown sugar

20. What does sturdy mean?

a. Long

b. Strong

c. Short

d. Wide

21. What does disperse mean?

a. Scatter

b. To form a ball

c. To stir

d. To beat

22. When can you stop stirring the nuts?

a. When the cookies are cooked.

b. When the nuts are evenly distributed.

c. When the nuts are added.

d. After the chocolate chips are added.

Questions 23 - 26 refer to the following passage.

Passage 5 - Frankenstein

Great God! What a scene has just taken place! I am yet dizzy with the remembrance of it. I hardly know whether I shall have the power to detail it; yet the tale which I have recorded would be incomplete without this final and wonderful catastrophe. I entered the cabin where lay the remains of my ill-fated and admirable friend. Over him hung a form which I cannot find words to describe—gigantic in stature, yet uncouth and distorted in its proportions. As he hung over the coffin, his face was concealed by long locks of ragged hair; but one vast hand was extended, in color and apparent texture like that of a mummy. When he heard the sound of my approach, he ceased to utter exclamations of grief and horror and sprung towards the window. Never did I behold a vision so horrible as his face, of such loathsome yet appalling hideousness. I shut my eyes involuntarily and endeavored to recollect what were my duties with regard to this destroyer. I called on him to stay.

He paused, looking on me with wonder, and again turning towards the lifeless form of his creator, he seemed to forget my presence, and every feature and gesture seemed instigated by the wildest rage of some uncontrollable passion.

"That is also my victim!" he exclaimed. "In his murder my crimes are consummated; the miserable series of my being is wound to its close! Oh, Frankenstein! Generous and self-devoted being! What does it avail that I now ask thee to pardon me? I, who irretrievably destroyed thee by destroying all thou lovedst. Alas! He is cold, he cannot answer me."

His voice seemed suffocated, and my first impulses, which had suggested to me the duty of obeying the dying request of my friend in destroying his enemy, were now suspended by a mixture of curiosity and compassion. I approached this tremendous being; I dared not again raise my eyes to his face, there was something so scaring and unearthly in his ugliness. I attempted to speak, but the words died away on my lips. The monster continued to utter wild and incoherent self-reproaches. At length I gathered resolution to address him in a pause of the tempest of his passion.

"Your repentance," I said, "is now superfluous. If you had listened to the voice of conscience and heeded the stings of remorse before you had urged your diabolical vengeance to this extremity, Frankenstein would yet have lived." [7]

23. Who is the "ill-fated and admirable friend" who is lying in the coffin?

    a. Frankenstein's monster

    b. Frankenstein

    c. Mary Shelley

    d. Unknown

24. Why is the speaker 'suspended" from following through on his duty to destroy the monster?

a. The way the monster looks

b. The monster's remorse

c. Curiosity and compassion

d. Fear the monster might kill him too

25. How does Frankenstein's monster destroy Frankenstein?

a. By killing Frankenstein

b. By letting himself be the monster everyone sees him as

c. By destroying everything Frankenstein loved

d. All of the above

26. When the Speaker says the monster's repentance is "superfluous, what does he mean?

a. That it is unnecessary and unused because Frankenstein is already dead and cannot hear him

b. That he accepts the repentance on behalf of Frankenstein

c. That the monster does not actually feel remorseful

d. That his repentance is unneeded because he did not do anything wrong

Questions 27 - 30 refer to the following passage.

Lowest Price Guarantee

Get it for less. Guaranteed!

ABC Electric will beat any advertised price by 10% of the difference.

1) If you find a lower advertised price, we will beat it by 10% of the difference.

2) If you find a lower advertised price within 30 days* of your purchase we will beat it by 10% of the difference.

3) If our own price is reduced within 30 days* of your purchase, bring in your receipt and we will refund the difference.

*14 days for computers, monitors, printers, laptops, tablets, cellular & wireless devices, home security products, projectors, camcorders, digital cameras, radar detectors, portable DVD players, DJ and pro-audio equipment, and air conditioners.

27. I bought a radar detector 15 days ago and saw an ad for the same model only cheaper. Can I get 10% of the difference refunded?

a. Yes. Since it is less than 30 days, you can get 10% of the difference refunded.

b. No. Since it is more than 14 days, you cannot get 10% of the difference re-funded.

c. It depends on the cashier.

d. Yes. You can get the difference refunded.

28. I bought a flat-screen TV for $500 10 days ago and found an advertisement for the same TV, at another store, on sale for $400. How much will ABC refund under this guarantee?

a. $100

b. $110

c. $10

d. $400

29. What is the purpose of this passage?

a. To inform

b. To educate

c. To persuade

d. To entertain

Questions 30 - 33 refer to the following passage.

Passage 6 - What Is Mardi Gras?

Mardi Gras is fast becoming one of the South's most famous and most celebrated holidays. The word Mardi Gras comes from the French and the literal translation is "Fat Tuesday." The holiday has also been called Shrove Tuesday, due to its associations with Lent. The purpose of Mardi Gras is to celebrate and enjoy before the Lenten season of fasting and repentance begins.

What originated by the French Explorers in New Orleans, Louisiana in the 17th century is now celebrated all over the world. Panama, Italy, Belgium and Brazil all host large scale Mardi Gras celebrations, and many smaller cities and towns celebrate this fun loving Tuesday as well. Usually held in February or early March, Mardi Gras is a day of extravagance, a day for people to eat, drink and be merry, to wear costumes, masks and to dance to jazz music.
The French explorers on the Mississippi River would be in shock today if they saw the opulence of the parades and floats that grace the New Orleans streets during Mardi Gras these days. Parades in New Orleans are divided by organizations. These are more commonly known as Krewes.

Being a member of a Krewe is quite a task because Krewes are responsible for overseeing the parades. Each Krewe's parade is ruled by a Mardi Gras "King and Queen." The role of the King and Queen is to "bestow" gifts on their adoring fans as the floats ride along the street. They throw doubloons, which is fake money and usually colored green, purple and gold, which are the colors of Mardi Gras. Beads in those color shades are also thrown and cups are thrown as well. Beads are by far the most popular souvenir of any Mardi Gras parade, with each spectator attempting to gather as many as possible.

30. The purpose of Mardi Gras is to

    a. Repent for a month.

    b. Celebrate in extravagant ways.

    c. Be a member of a Krewe.

    d. Explore the Mississippi.

31. From reading the passage we can infer that "Kings and Queens"

    a. Have to be members of a Krewe.

    b. Have to be French.

    c. Have to know how to speak French.

    d. Have to give away their own money.

32. Which group of people first began to hold Mardi Gras celebrations?

    a. Settlers from Italy

    b. Members of Krewes

    c. French explorers

    d. Belgium explorers

33. In the context of the passage, what does the word spectator most nearly mean?

    a. Someone who participates actively

    b. Someone who watches the parade's action

    c. Someone on one of the parade floats

    d. Someone who does not celebrate Mardi Gras

Questions 34 - 35 refer to the following passage.

Passage 7 - Peter Pan

Author: James M. Barrie

All children, except one, grow up. They soon know that they will grow up, and the way Wendy knew was this. One day when she was two years old she was playing in a garden, and she plucked another flower and ran with it to her mother. I suppose she must have looked rather delightful, for Mrs. Darling put her hand to her heart and cried, "Oh, why can't you remain like this for ever!" This was all that passed between them on the subject, but henceforth Wendy knew that she must grow up. You always know after you are two. Two is the beginning of the end.

Of course they lived at 14 [their house number on their street], and until Wendy came her mother was the chief one. She was a lovely lady, with a romantic mind and such a sweet mocking mouth. Her romantic mind was like the tiny boxes, one within the other, that come from the puzzling East, however many you discover there is always one more; and her sweet mocking mouth had one kiss on it that Wendy could never get, though there it was, perfectly conspicuous in the right-hand corner.

The way Mr. Darling won her was this: the many gentlemen who had been boys when she was a girl discovered simultaneously that they loved her, and they all ran to her house to propose to her except Mr. Darling, who took a cab and nipped in first, and so he got her. He got all of her, except the innermost box and the kiss. He never knew about the box, and in time he gave up trying for the kiss. Wendy thought Napoleon could have got it, but I can picture him trying, and then going off in a passion, slamming the door.

34. The author's description of Mrs. Darling's "sweet mocking mouth" implies:

    a. While pretty, Mrs. Darling frequently chides others.

    b. Although subject to slight disfigurement, Mrs. Darling's mouth is still pleasant in appearance.

    c. Mrs. Darling uses her words to get her way.

    d. Mrs. Darling is a loving woman, yet she does not wholly give her love away.

35. Overall, from this passage you can infer that Mrs. Darling:

    a. Is a dominant, complex woman.

    b. Accidentally denies those around her.

    c. Is artistic and absent-minded.

    d. Has a troubled marriage.

Section II – Math

1. Richard gives 's' amount of salary to each of his 'n' employees weekly. If he has 'x' amount of money, how many days he can employ these 'n' employees.

    a. $sx/7n$

    b. $7x/nx$

    c. $nx/7s$

    d. $7x/ns$

2. Translate the following into an equation: Five greater than 3 times a number.

    a. 3X + 5

    b. 5X + 3

    c. (5 + 3)X

    d. 5(3 + X)

3. What number is MMXIII?

    a. 2010

    b. 1990

    c. 2013

    d. 2012

4. Solve for x, when 5x + 21 = 66.

    a. 19

    b. 9

    c. 15

    d. 5

5. Write 765.3682 to the nearest 1000th.

    a. 765.368

    b. 765.36

    c. 765.3682

    d. 765.3

6. If Lynn can type a page in p minutes, what portion of the page can she do in 5 minutes?

    a. p/5

    b. p - 5

    c. p + 5

    d. 5/p

7. If Sally can paint a house in 4 hours, and John can paint the same house in 6 hours, how long will it take for both of to paint a house?

    a. 2 hours and 24 minutes

    b. 3 hours and 12 minutes

    c. 3 hours and 44 minutes

    d. 4 hours and 10 minutes

8. Employees of a discount appliance store receive an additional 20% off the lowest price on any item. If an employee purchases a dishwasher during a 15% off sale, how much will he pay if the dishwasher originally cost $450?

    a. $280.90

    b. $287.00

    c. $292.50

    d. $306.00

9. The sale price of a car is $12,590, which is 20% off the original price. What is the original price?

    a. $14,310.40

    b. $14,990.90

    c. $15,108.00

    d. $15,737.50

10. Express 25% as a fraction.

    a. 1/4

    b. 7/40

    c. 6/25

    d. 8/28

11. Express 125% as a decimal.

    a. .125

    b. 12.5

    c. 1.25

    d. 125

12. Express 24/56 as a reduced common fraction.

    a. 4/9

    b. 4/11

    c. 3/7

    d. 3/8

13. Express 71/1000 as a decimal.

    a. .71

    b. .0071

    c. .071

    d. 7.1

14. What number is in the ten thousandths place in 1.7389?

    a. 1

    b. 8

    c. 9

    d. 3

15. Simplify 6 3/5 – 4 4/5

  a. 1 4/5

  b. 2 3/5

  c. 2 9/5

  d. 1 1/5

16. The physician ordered 100 mg Ibuprofen/kg of body weight; on hand is 230 mg/tablet. The child weighs 50 lb. How many tablets will you give?

  a. 10 tablets

  b. 5 tablets

  c. 1 tablet

  d. 12 tablets

17. In wa local election at polling station A, 945 voters cast their vote out of 1270 registered voters. At polling station B, 860 cast their vote out of 1050 registered voters and at station C, 1210 cast their vote out of 1440 registered voters. What is the total turnout from all three polling stations?

  a. 70%

  b. 74%

  c. 76%

  d. 80%

18. The physician ordered 600 mg ibuprofen; the pharmacy stocks 200 mg per tablet. How many tablets will you give?

  a. 3.5 tablets

  b. 2 tablets

  c. 5 tablets

  d. 3 tablets

19. The manager of a weaving factory estimates that if 10 machines run at 100% efficiency for 8 hours, they will produce 1450 meters of cloth. Due to some technical problems, 4 machines run of 95% efficiency and the remaining 6 at 90% efficiency. How many meters of cloth can these machines will produce in 8 hours?

    a. 1334 meters

    b. 1310 meters

    c. 1300 meters

    d. 1285 meters

20. Convert 60 feet to inches.

    a. 700 inches

    b. 600 inches

    c. 720 inches

    d. 1,800 inches

21. A box contains 7 black pencils and 28 blue ones. What is the ratio between the black and blue pens?

    a. 1:4

    b. 2:7

    c. 1:8

    d. 1:9

22. Convert 100 millimeters to centimeters.

    a. 10 centimeters

    b. 1,000 centimeters

    c. 1100 centimeters

    d. 50 centimeters

23. Convert 3 gallons to quarts.

  a. 15 quarts

  b. 6 quarts

  c. 12 quarts

  d. 32 quarts

24. A map uses a scale of 1:2,000 How much distance on the ground is 5.2 inches on the map if the scale is in inches?

  a. 100,400

  b. 10, 500

  c. 10,440

  d. 10,400

25. 0.05 ml. =

  a. 50 liters

  b. 0.00005 liters

  c. 5 liters

  d. 0.0005 liters

26. X% of 120 = 30. Solve for X.

  a. 15

  b. 12

  c. 4

  d. 25

27. Smith and Simon are playing a card game. Smith will win if a card drawn from a deck of 52 is either 7 or a diamond, and Simon will win if the drawn card is an even number. Which statement is more likely to be correct?

    a. Smith will win more games.

    b. Simon will win more games.

    c. They have same winning probability.

    d. A decision cannot be made from the provided data.

28. Convert .45 meters to centimeters

    a. 45

    b. 450

    c. 4.5

    d. .45

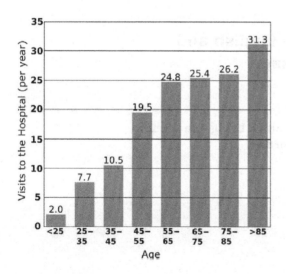

29. Consider the graph above.

How many hospital visits per year does a person aged 85 or more make?

    a. 26.2

    b. 31.3

    c. More than 31.3

    d. A decision cannot be made from this graph.

30. Based on this graph, how many visits per year do you expect a person that is 95 or older to make?

    a. 31.3 or more

    b. Less than 31.3

    c. 31.3

    d. A decision cannot be made from this graph.

Section III – English and Language Usage

1. Elaine promised to bring the camera _____ at the mall yesterday.

    a. by me

    b. with me

    c. at me

    d. to me

2. Last night, he _____ the sleeping bag down beside my mattress.

    a. lay

    b. laid

    c. lain

    d. has laid

3. I would have bought the shirt for you if

    a. I had known you liked it.

    b. I have known you liked it.

    c. I would know you liked it.

    d. I know you liked it.

4. Many believers still hope _____ proof of the existence of ghosts.

    a. two find

    b. to find

    c. to found

    d. to have been found

5. Choose the sentence with the correct grammar.

    a. The court summons was placed on his desk

    b. The court summons are placed on his desk

    c. The court summons were placed on his desk

    d. None of the above

6. To _____, Anne was on time for her math class.

    a. everybody's surprise

    b. every body's surprise

    c. everybodys surprise

    d. everybodys' surprise

7. As an added bonus, we got to see the orchestra warm up.

What part of this sentence is redundant?

    a. Added

    b. Bonus

    c. Warm up

    d. None of the above

8. If he _____ the textbook like he was supposed to, he would have known what was on the test.

    a. will have read

    b. shouldn't have read

    c. would have read

    d. had read

9. Following the tornado, telephone poles _____ all over the street.

    a. laid

    b. lied

    c. were lying

    d. were laying

10. In Edgar Allen Poe's _____ Edgar Allen Poe describes a man with a guilty conscience.

    a. short story, "The Tell-Tale Heart,"

    b. short story The Tell-Tale Heart,

    c. short story, The Tell-Tale Heart

    d. short story. "the Tell-Tale Heart,"

11. Billboards are considered an important part of advertising for big business, _____ by their critics.

    a. but, an eyesore;

    b. but, " an eyesore,"

    c. but an eyesore

    d. but-an eyesore-

12. I can never remember how to use those two common words, "sell," meaning to trade a product for money, or _____ meaning an event where products are traded for less money than usual.

    a. sale-

    b. "sale,"

    c. "sale

    d. "to sale,"

13. Choose the sentence with the correct grammar.

    a. Neither the teacher nor the students is left in class.

    b. Neither the teacher nor the students was left in class.

    c. Neither the teacher nor the students are left in class.

    d. None of the above.

14. The class just finished reading _____ a short story by Carl Stephenson about a plantation owner's battle with army ants.

    a. -"Leinengen versus the Ants,"

    b. Leinengen versus the Ants,

    c. "Leinengen versus the Ants,"

    d. Leinengen versus the Ants

15. After the car was fixed, it _____ again.

    a. ran good

    b. ran well

    c. would have run well

    d. ran more well

16. "Where does the sun go during the _____ asked little Kathy.

    a. night,"

    b. night"?,

    c. night,?"

    d. night?"

17. Choose the correct spelling.

    a. conscentious

    b. conscientios

    c. conscientious

    d. consceintious

18. I have finished studying for today.

What type of sentence is this?

    a. Imperative

    b. Interrogative

    c. Exclamatory

    d. Declarative

19. Which of the following sentences contains a redundant phrase?

    a. I haven't seen her for ages.

    b. My suitcase is books all the way to Amsterdam.

    c. The end result was very disappointing.

    d. None of the above.

20. Choose the correct sentence.

    a. Their only employee with a nose ring is a young man named Daniel.

    b. Their only employee is a young man named Daniel with a nose ring.

    c. Their only employee is a young man with a nose ring named Daniel.

    d. A and C are correct.

21. Choose the sentence with the correct grammar.

    a. Everyone are to wear a black tie.

    b. Everyone have to wear a black tie.

    c. Everyone has to wear a black tie.

    d. None of the above.

22. Choose the correct spelling.

    a. leisuire

    b. lesure

    c. lesure

    d. lcisurc

Practice the TEAS®

23. Choose the correct spelling.

   a. pigeone

   b. pigoen

   c. pigeon

   d. pidgeon

24. Choose the correct spelling.

   a. odyessy

   b. odeyssey

   c. odysey

   d. odyssey

25. Choose the sentence with the correct grammar.

   a. The salmon has been cooked.

   b. The salmon have been cooked.

   c. Both of the above.

   d. None of the above.

26. This is absolutely incredible _____

   a. !

   b. .

   c. :

   d. ;

27. Watch out for the broken glass _____

   a. .

   b. ?

   c. ,

   d. !

28. I still don't know exactly. That isn't _____ evidence.

    a. Undeterred

    b. Unrelenting

    c. Unfortunate

    d. Conclusive

29. He walked all the way downtown.

What is the simple subject of this sentence?

    a. He

    b. Walked

    c. Downtown

    d. All the way

30. He could manipulate the coins in his fingers very

    a. Brazenly

    b. Eloquently

    c. Boisterously

    d. Deftly

Section IV – Science

1. Which of the following is not true

    a. Genotypes are inherited information

    b. Phenotypes are inherited information

    c. Phenotypes are observed behavior

    d. Phenotypes include an organisms development

2. Electrons play a critical role in

    a. Electricity

    b. Magnetism

    c. Thermal conductivity

    d. All of the above

3. An idea concerning a phenomena and possible explanations for that phenomena is a/an

    a. Theory

    b. Experiment

    c. Inference

    d. Hypothesis

4. Define chromosomes.

    a. Structures in a cell nucleus that carry genetic material.

    b. Consist of thousands of DNA strands.

    c. Total 46 in a normal human cell.

    d. All of the above

5. What is one of the best known disorders that attack the immune system?

    a. Rabies

    b. HIV

    c. Lung cancer

    d. Muscular dystrophy

6. Which disease of the circulatory system is one of the most frequent causes of death in North America?

    a. The cold

    b. Pneumonia

    c. Arthritis

    d. Heart disease

7. Which of the following describes a plasma membrane?

    a. Lipids with embedded proteins

    b. An outer lipid layer and an inner lipid layer

    c. Proteins embedded in lipid bilayer

    d. Altering protein and lipid layers

8. What is the difference between Strong Nuclear Force and Weak Nuclear Force?

    a. The Strong Nuclear Force is an attractive force that binds protons and neutrons and maintains the structure of the nucleus, and the Weak Nuclear Force is responsible for the radioactive beta decay and other subatomic reactions.

    b. The Strong Nuclear Force is responsible for the radioactive beta decay and other subatomic reactions, and the Weak Nuclear Force is an attractive force that binds protons and neutrons and maintains the structure of the nucleus.

    c. The Weak Nuclear Force is feeble and the Strong Nuclear Force is robust.

    d. The Strong Nuclear Force is a negative force that releases protons and neutrons and threatens the structure of the nucleus, and the Weak Nuclear Force is an attractive force that binds protons and neutrons and maintains the structure of the nucleus.

9. What type of research studies the quality, type or components of a group, substance, or mixture?

    a. Quantitative

    b. Dependent

    c. Scientific

    d. Qualitative

10. Adaptation is

    a. A trait that has evolved by natural selection.

    b. A trait that has been bred by artificial selection.

    c. A trait that has no function in an organism.

    d. None of the above.

11. Describe a pH indicator.

    a. A pH indicator measures hydrogen ions in a solution and show pH on a color scale.

    b. A pH indicator measures oxygen ions in a solution and show pH on a color scale.

    c. A pH indicator many different types of ions in a solution and shows pH on a color scale.

    d. None of the above.

12. What is the earth's primary source of energy?

    a. Water

    b. The sun

    c. Electromagnetic radiation

    d. Weak nuclear force

13. What type of research is to determine the relationship between one thing (an independent variable) and another (a dependent or outcome variable) in a population?

    a. Qualitative

    b. Quantitative

    c. Independent

    d. Scientific

14. What can accept a hydrogen ion and can react with fats to form soaps?

    a. Acid

    b. Salt

    c. Base

    d. Foundation

15. Which gene, whose presence as a single copy, controls the expression of a trait?

    a. Principal gene

    b. Latent gene

    c. Recessive gene

    d. Dominant gene

16. Within taxonomy, plants and animals are considered two basic

    a. Families

    b. Kingdoms

    c. Domains

    d. Genus

**17. Organisms grouped into the _____ Kingdom in-
clude all unicellular organisms lacking a definite cellular
arrangement such as _____ and _____.**

    a. Fungi, bacteria, algae

    b. Protista, bacteria, amphibian

    c. Protista, bacteria, algae

    d. Plantae, bacteria, algae

**18. What is a common digestive affliction most people
suffer at one time or
other?**

    a. Stomach cancer

    b. Ulceritis

    c. Indigestion

    d. The flu

**19. What are the biochemical and biophysical activities
that all living systems must be able to carry out to maintain life?**

    a. Life sequences

    b. Life expectancies

    c. Life cycles

    d. Life functions

**20. What disease of the circulatory system is often mis-
taken for a heart attack?**

    a. Cardiac arrest

    b. High blood pressure

    c. Angina

    d. Acid reflux

21. Define a biological class.

a. A collection of similar or like living entities.

b. Two or more animals in a group, all having the same parent.

c. All animals sharing the same living environment.

d. All plant life that share the same physical properties.

22. What type of foods that stay in the stomach the longest?

a. Fats

b. Proteins

c. Carbohydrates

d. Vitamins

23. What is a graphical description of feeding relationships among species in an ecological community?

a. Food web

b. Food chain

c. Food network

d. Food sequence

24. What is the diagram that is used to predict an outcome of a particular cross or breeding experiment?

a. Genetic puzzle

b. Genome project

c. Hybrid theorem

d. Punnett square

25. Which, if any, of the following statements about prokaryotic cells is false?

a. Prokaryotic cells include such organisms as E. coli and Streptococcus.

b. Prokaryotic cells lack internal membranes and organelles.

c. Prokaryotic cells break down food using cellular respiration and fermentation.

d. All of these statements are true.

26. What is the process of converting observed phenomena into data is called?

a. Calculation

b. Measurement

c. Valuation

d. Estimation

27. The mass number of an atom is

a. The total number of particles that make it up.

b. The total weight of an atom.

c. The total mass of an atom.

d. None of the above.

28. What is sublimation?

a. A phase transition from liquid to gas.

b. A phase transition from solid to gas.

c. A phase transition from gas to liquid.

d. A phase transition from gas to solid.

29. How is exhalation accomplished?

a. By the abdominal muscles

b. By the chest muscles

c. By the esophagus

d. By the nasal passageway

30. What three processes are involved in cell division of Eukaryotic cells?

a. Meiosis, mitosis, and interphase

b. Meiosis, mitosis, and interphase

c. Mitosis, kinematisis, and interphase

d. Mitosis, cytokinesis, and interphase

31. Describe genotypes.

a. The genetic makeup, as distinguished from the physical appearance, of an organism or a group of organisms.

b. The combination of alleles located on homologous chromosomes that determines a specific characteristic or trait.

c. Is the inheritable information carried by all living organisms.

d. All of the above.

32. What does the respiratory system primarily oxygenate?

a. The brain

b. The limbs

c. The heart

d. The blood

33. What chain of nucleotides plays an important role in the creation of new proteins?

a. Deoxyribonucleic acid (DNA) is a chain of nucleotides that plays an important role in the creation of new proteins.

b. Ribonucleic acid (RNA) is a chain of nucleotides that plays an important role in the creation of new proteins.

c. There are no chains of nucleotides that play a role in the creation of proteins.

d. None of the above.

34. A practical test designed with the intention that its results will be relevant to a particular theory or set of theories is a/an

a. Experiment

b. Practicum

c. Theory

d. Design

35. Strong chemical bonds include

a. Dipole - dipole interactions.

b. Hydrogen bonding.

c. Covalent or ionic bonds.

d. None of the above.

36. What is the process that the immune system adapts over time to be more efficient in recognizing pathogens?

a. Acquired immunity

b. AIDS

c. Pathogens

d. Acquired deficiency

37. What is a group of tissues that perform a specific function or group of functions?

    a. System

    b. Tissue

    c. Group

    d. Organ

38. What is the measure of an experiment's ability to yield the same or compatible results in different clinical experiments or statistical trials?

    a. Variability

    b. Validity

    c. Control measure

    d. Reliability

39. Describe each chemical element in the periodic table.

    a. Each chemical element has a unique atomic number representing the number of electrons in its nucleus.

    b. Each chemical element has a varying atomic number depending on the number of protons in its nucleus.

    c. Each chemical element has a unique atomic number representing the number of protons in its nucleus.

    d. None of the above.

40. The immune system is

    a. The system that expels waste from the body.

    b. The system that expels carbon dioxide from the body.

    c. The system that protects the body from disease and infection.

    d. The system that circulates blood through the body.

41. The binding membrane of an animal cell is called

    a. The biological membrane.

    b. The cell coat.

    c. The unit membrane.

    d. The plasma membrane.

42. Define organelles.

    a. A protein in a cell

    b. An enzyme in a cell

    c. A specialized subunit of a cell with a specific function

    d. A cell membrane

43. A solution with a pH value of less than 7 is

    a. Acid solution.

    b. Base solution.

    c. Neutral pH solution.

    d. None of the above.

44. Is a catalyst changed by a reaction?

    a. Yes

    b. No

    c. It may be changed depending on the other chemicals.

45. What is the prediction that an observed difference is due to chance alone and not due to a systematic cause? This hypothesis is tested by statistical analysis, and either accepted or rejected.

    a. Null hypothesis

    b. Hypothesis

    c. Control

    d. Variable

46. In science, industry, and statistics, the _____ of a measurement system is the degree of closeness of measurements of a quantity to its actual (true) value.

a. Mistake

b. Uncertainty

c. Accuracy

d. Error

47. What is a more common name for the circulatory system disease known as hypertension?

a. Anemia

b. High blood pressure

c. Angina

d. Cardiac arrest

48. Given a normal distribution, what is the difference between the maximum value and the minimum value?

a. Distribution

b. Range

c. Mode

d. Median

Quick Reference Answer Key

Part I - Reading

1. A
2. C
3. D
4. A
5. B
6. C
7. B
8. A
9. D
10. B
11. A
12. A
13. C
14. C
15. A
16. B
17. A
18. B
19. A
20. B
21. A
22. B
23. B
24. C
25. D
26. A
27. B
28. B
29. C
30. B
31. A
32. C
33. B
34. D
35. A

Section II – Math

1. D
2. A
3. C
4. B
5. A
6. D
7. A
8. D
9. D
10. A
11. C
12. C
13. C
14. C
15. A
16. A
17. D
18. D
19. A
20. C
21. A
22. A
23. C
24. D
25. B
26. D
27. B
28. A
29. A
30. A

Section III – English and Language Usage

1. D
2. A
3. A

4. B
5. A
6. A
7. A
8. D
9. C
10. A
11. C
12. B
13. C
14. C
15. B
16. D
17. C
18. D
19. C
20. D
21. C
22. D
23. C
24. D
25. C
26. A
27. D
28. D
29. A
30. D

Section IV – Science

1. B
2. D
3. D
4. D
5. B
6. D
7. C
8. A
9. D
10. A
11. A

12. B
13. B
14. C
15. D
16. B
17. C
18. C
19. D
20. C
21. A
22. A
23. A
24. D
25. D
26. B
27. A
28. B
29. A
30. D
31. D
32. D
33. B
34. A
35. C
36. A
37. D
38. D
39. C
40. C
41. D
42. C
43. A
44. B
45. A
46. C
47. B
48. B

Answer Key with Explanations

1. A
Choice B is incorrect; the author did not express their opinion on the subject matter. Choice C is incorrect, the author was not trying to prove a point.

2. C
Choice C is correct; historians believe it was brutal and bloody. Choice A is incorrect; there is no consensus that the Crusades achieved great things. Choice B is incorrect; it did not stabilize the Holy Lands. Choice D is incorrect, some historians do believe this was the purpose but not all historians.

3. D
The feudal system led to infighting. Choice A is incorrect, it had the opposite effect. Choice B is incorrect, though this is a good answer, it is not the best answer. The Church asked for volunteers not the Feudal Lords. Choice C is incorrect, it did have an effect on the Crusades.

4. A
Saracen was a generic term for Muslims widely used in Europe during the later medieval era.

5. B
This warranty does not cover a product that you have tried to fix yourself. From paragraph two, "This limited warranty does not cover ... any unauthorized disassembly, repair, or modification. "

6. C
ABC Electric could either replace or repair the fan, provided the other conditions are met. ABC Electric has the option to repair or replace.

7. B
The warranty does not cover a stove damaged in a flood. From the passage, "This limited warranty does not cover any damage to the product from improper installation, accident, abuse, misuse, natural disaster, insufficient or excessive

electrical supply, abnormal mechanical or environmental conditions."

A flood is an "abnormal environmental condition," and a natural disaster, so it is not covered.

8. A
A missing part is an example of defective workmanship. This is an error made in the manufacturing process. A defective part is not considered workmanship.

9. D
This question tests the reader's summarization skills. The other choices A, B, and C focus on portions of the second paragraph that are too narrow and do not relate to the specific portion of text in question. The complexity of the sentence may mislead students into selecting one of these answers, but rearranging or restating the sentence will lead the reader to the correct answer. In addition, choice A makes an assumption that may or may not be true about the intentions of the company, choice B focuses on one product rather than the idea of the products, and choice C makes an assumption about women that may or may not be true and is not supported by the text.

10. B
This question tests reader's attention to detail. If a reader selects A, he or she may have picked up on the use of the word "debate" and assumed, very logically, that the two are at odds because they are fighting; however, this is simply not supported in the text. Choice C also uses very specific quotes from the text, but it rearranges and gives them false meaning. The artists want to elevate their creations above the creations of other artists, thereby showing that they are "creative" and "innovative." Similarly, choice D takes phrases straight from the text and rearranges and confuses them. The artists are described as wanting to be "creative, innovative, individual people," not the women.

11. A
This question tests reader's vocabulary and summarization skills. This phrase, used by the author, may seem flippant and dismissive if readers focus on the word "whatever" and

misinterpret it as a popular, colloquial term. In this way, choices B and C may mislead the reader to selecting one of them by including the terms "unimportant" and "stupid," respectively. Choice D is a similar misreading, but doesn't make sense when the phrase is at the beginning of the passage and the entire passage is on media messages. Choice A is literally and contextually appropriate, and the reader can understand that the author would like to keep the introduction focused on the topic the passage is going to discuss.

12. A
This question tests a reader's inference skills. The extreme use of the word "all" in choice B suggests that every single advertising company are working to be approachable, and while this is not only unlikely, the text specifically states that "more" companies have done this, signifying that they have not all participated, even if it's a possibility that they may some day. The use of the limiting word "only" in choice C lends that answer similar problems; women are still buying from companies who do not care about this message, or those companies would not be in business, and the passage specifies that "many" women are worried about media messages, but not all. Readers may find choice D logical, especially if they are looking to make an inference, and while this may be a possibility, the passage does not suggest or discuss this happening. Choice A is correct based on specifically because of the relation between "still working" in the answer and "will hopefully" and the extensive discussion on companies struggles, which come only with progress, in the text.

13. C
This question tests the reader's summarization skills. The entire passage is leading up to the idea that the president of the US may not have had grounds to assert his Fourteen Points when other countries had lost so much. Choice A is pretty directly inferred by the text, but it does not adequately summarize what the entire passage is trying to communicate. Choice B may also be inferred by the passage when it says that the war is "imminent," but it does not represent the entire message, either. The passage does seem to be in praise of FDR, or at least in respect of him, but it does not in any way claim that he is the smartest president, nor does this represent the many other points included. Choice C is

then the obvious answer, and most directly relates to the closing sentences which it rewords.

14. C
This question tests the reader's attention to detail. The passage does state that choices A and B are true, and while those statements are in proximity to the explanation for why the war started, they are not the reason given. Choice D is a mix up of words used in the passage, which says that the largest powers were in play but not that this fact somehow started the war. The passage does make a direct statement that a domino effect started the war, supporting choice C as the correct answer.

15. A
This question tests the reader's understanding of functions in writing. Throughout the passage, it states that leaders of other nations were hesitant to accept generous or peaceful terms because of the grievances of the war, and the great loss of life was chief among these. While the passage does touch on the devastation of deadly weapons (B), the use of this raw, emotional fact serves a much larger purpose, and the focus of the passage is not the weapons. While readers may indeed consider who lost the most soldiers (C) when, so many countries were involved and the inequalities of loss are mentioned in the passage, there is no discussion of this in the passage. Choice D is related to A, but choice A is more direct and relates more to the passage.

16. B
This question tests the reader's vocabulary skills. Choice A may seem appealing to readers because it is phonetically similar to "catalyzed," but the two are not related in any other way. Choice C makes sense in context, but if plugged in to the sentence creates a redundancy that doesn't make sense. Choice D does also not make sense contextually, even if the reader may consider that funds were needed to create more weaponry, especially if it was advanced.

17. A
Victoria is about 5 miles from Burnaby.

18. B
The Village Hall is about 5 miles from Victoria.

19. A
The correct order of ingredients is brown sugar, baking soda and chocolate chips.

20. B
Sturdy: strong, solid in structure or person. In context, Stir in chocolate chips by hand with a *sturdy* wooden spoon.

21. A
Disperse: to scatter in different directions or break up. In context, Stir until the chocolate chips and nuts are evenly *dispersed*.

22. B
You can stop stirring the nuts when they are evenly distributed. From the passage, "Stir until the chocolate chips and nuts are evenly dispersed."

23. B
Choice A is incorrect as the Monster killed Frankenstein, not the other way around. Choice B is correct, Frankenstein is dead. Choice C is incorrect - Mary Shelley is the author. Choice D is incorrect, the person is called Frankenstein.

24. C
The speaker 'suspended' from following through on his duty to destroy the monster due to curiosity and compassion. The other choices may seem reasonable, but are not explicitly given in the passage.

25. D
All the choices are correct.   Frankenstein's monster destroys Frankenstein by

   a. By killing Frankenstein

   b. By letting himself be the monster everyone sees him as

   c. By destroying everything Frankenstein loved

26. A
Superfluous means unnecessary. Looking at the context of the word as it is used in the passage:

"Your repentance," I said, "is now superfluous. If you had listened to the voice of conscience and heeded the stings of remorse before you had urged your diabolical vengeance to this extremity, Frankenstein would yet have lived."

27. B
The time limit for radar detectors is 14 days. Since you made the purchase 15 days ago, you do not qualify for the guarantee.

28. B
Since you made the purchase 10 days ago, you are covered by the guarantee. Since it is an advertised price at a different store, ABC Electric will "beat" the price by 10% of the difference, which is,

$500 - 400 = 100$ – difference in price

$100 \times 10\% = \$10$ – 10% of the difference

The advertised lower price is $400. ABC will beat this price by 10% so they will refund $100 + 10 = $110.

29. C
The purpose of this passage is to persuade.

30. B
The correct answer can be found in the fourth sentence of the first paragraph.

Choice A is incorrect because repenting begins the day AFTER Mardi Gras. Choice C is incorrect because you can celebrate Mardi Gras without being a member of a Krewe.

Choice D is incorrect because exploration does not play any role in a modern Mardi Gras celebration.

31. A
The second sentence is the last paragraph states that Krewes are led by the Kings and Queens. Therefore, you must

have to be part of a Krewe to be its King or its Queen.

Choice B is incorrect because it never states in the passage that only people from France can be Kings and Queen of Mardi Gras

Choice C is incorrect because the passage says nothing about having to speak French.

Choice D is incorrect because the passage does state that the Kings and Queens throw doubloons, which is fake money.

32. C
The first sentences of BOTH the 2nd and 3rd paragraphs mention that French explorers started this tradition in New Orleans.
Choices A, B and D are incorrect because they are just names of cities or countries listed in the 2nd paragraph.

33. B
In the final paragraph the word spectator is used to describe people who are watching the parade and catching cups, beads and doubloons.
Choices A and C are incorrect because we know the people who participate are part of Krewes. People who work the floats and parades are also part of Krewes

Choice D is incorrect because the passage makes no mention of people who do not celebrate Mardi Gras.

34. D
There is no concrete evidence of choices A, B, or C. Choice D is therefore the best answer, and the passage supports the notion that her mouth possess a special kiss that neither her daughter nor husband can attain, and in this way her mouth seems to mock them.

35. A
Choice A is the best-supported choice: The narrator notes, "Until Wendy came, her mother was the chief one," and further describes Mrs. Darling as a woman who will not compromise. Both Mr. Darling and Wendy are seemingly unable to access the full extent of Mrs. Darling's affection. The description of Mrs. Darling's mind as "like the tiny

boxes, one within the other, that come from the puzzling East" suggests she is a woman with many layers, is impossible to fully understand, and to this end has even a foreign quality to her. B is incorrect as nothing about her denial of her husband or daughter appears to be accidental. Choice C's "absent-minded" descriptor could be reasonable, yet "romantic" is not in this case the same as "artistic", and there is no evidence of Mrs. Darling's artistic ability. Again, in light of Mr. Darling giving up on the elusive kiss, choice D could be reasonable, however there is nothing to suggest a serious problem is present in the matrimony. Nothing

suggests Mrs. Darling is indecisive, choice E is incorrect.

Section II – Math
1. D
We understand that each of the n employees earn s amount of salary weekly. This means that one employee earns s salary weekly. So; Richard has ns amount of money to employ n employees for a week.

We are asked to find the number of days n employees can be employed with x amount of money. We can do simple direct proportion:

If Richard can employ n employees for 7 days with ns amount of money,

   Richard can employ n employees for y days with x amount of money ... y is the number of days we need to find.

We can do cross multiplication:

$y = (x \cdot 7)/(ns)$

$y = 7x/ns$

2. A
Five greater than 3 times a number.
5 + 3 times a number.
3X + 5

3. C
MMXIII is 2013. 1,000 + 1,000 + 10 + 1 + 1 + 1.

4. B
5b + 21 = 66, 5b = 66 – 21 = 45, 5b = 45, b = 45/5 = 9

5. A
The number is 51.738. The last digit, in the 1,000th place, 2, is less than 5, so it is discarded. Answer = 765.368.

6. D
This is a simple direct proportion problem:
If Lynn can type 1 page in p minutes,

   she can type x pages in 5 minutes

We do cross multiplication: x•p = 5•1

Then,

x = 5/p

7. A
This is an inverse ration problem.

1/x = 1/a + 1/b where a is the time Sally can paint a house, b is the time John can paint a house, x is the time Sally and John can together paint a house.

So,

1/x = 1/4 + 1/6 ... We use the least common multiple in the denominator that is 24:

1/x = 6/24 + 4/24

1/x = 10/24

x = 24/10

x = 2.4 hours.

In other words; 2 hours + 0.4 hours = 2 hours + 0.4•60 minutes

= 2 hours 24 minutes

8. D
The cost of the dishwasher = $450

15% discount amount = 450•15/100 = $67.5

The discounted price = 450 – 67.5 = $382.5

20% additional discount amount on lowest price = 382.5•20/100 = $76.5

So, the final discounted price = 382.5 - 76.5 = $306.00

9. D
Original price = x,
80/100 = 12590/X,
80X = 1259000,
X = 15,737.50.

10. A
25% = 25/100 = 1/4

11. C
125/100 = 1.25

12. C
24/56 = 3/7 (divide numerator and denominator by 8)

13. C
Converting a fraction into a decimal – divide the numerator by the denominator – so 71/1000 = .071. Dividing by 1000 moves the decimal point 3 places to the left.

14. C
9 is in the ten thousandths place in 1.7389, which is 4 places to the right of the decimal point.

15. A
(6-4) (3/5 – 4/5) = 2 (3-4/5) = since 3 is less than 4, we would have to subtract 1 from the whole number besides the fraction, therefore 1 4/5

16. A
Step 1: Set up the formula to calculate the dose to be given in mg as per weight of the child:-
Dose ordered X Weight in Kg = Dose to be given
Step 2: 100 mg X 23 kg = 2300 mg
(Convert 50 lb to Kg, 1 lb = 0.4536 kg, hence 50 lb = 50 X 0.4536 = 22.68 kg approx. 23 kg)
2300 mg/230 mg X 1 tablet/1 = 2300/230 = 10 tablets

17. D
To find the total turnout in all three polling stations, we need to proportion the number of voters to the number of all registered voters.

Number of total voters = 945 + 860 + 1210 = 3015

Number of total registered voters = 1270 + 1050 + 1440 = 3760

Percentage turnout over all three polling stations
= 3015 * 100/3760 = 80.19%

Checking the answers, we round 80.19 to the nearest whole number: 80%

18. D
600 mg/ 200 mg X 1 tablet/1 = 600/200 = 3 tablets

19. A
At 100% efficiency 1 machine produces 1450/10 = 145 m of cloth.

At 95% efficiency, 4 machines produce 4•145•95/100 = 551 m of cloth.

At 90% efficiency, 6 machines produce 6•145•90/100 = 783 m of cloth.

Total cloth produced by all 10 machines = 551 + 783 = 1334 m

Since the information provided and the question are based on 8 hours, we did not need to use time to reach the answer.

20. C
1 foot = 12 inches, 60 feet = 60 x 12 = 720 inches.

21. A
The ratio between black and blue pens is 7 to 28 or 7:28.
Bring to the lowest terms by dividing both sides by 7 gives
1:4.

22. A
1 millimeter = 10 centimeter, 100 millimeter = 100/10 = 10
centimeters.

23. C
1 gallon = 4 quarts, 3 gallons = 3 x 4 = 12 quarts.

24. D
1 inch on map = 2,000 inches on ground. So, 5.2 inches on
map = 5.2•2,000 = 10,400 inches on ground.

25. B
There are 1000 ml in a liter. 0.05/1000 = 0.00005 liters.

26. D
X% of 120 = 30,
X/100 = 30/120
So X = 30/120 x 100/1
3000/120 = 300/12
X = 25

27. B
There are 52 cards in total. Smith has 16 cards in which
he can win. Therefore, his probability of winning in a single
game will be 16/52. Simon has 20 winning cards so his
probability of winning in single draw is 20/52.

28. A
There are 100 centimeters in a meter, so 100 X .45 meters =
45.

29. A
Based on this graph, a person that is 85 or older will make
26.2 visits to the hospital every year.

30. A
A person aged 95 or older would make 31.3 or more visits.

Section III – English and Language Usage

1. D
The preposition "to" is correct. 'To' here means give.

2. A
"Lie" means to recline, and does not take an object. "lay" means to place and does take an object.

3. A
Past unreal conditional. Takes the form,
[If ... Past Perfect ..., ... would have + past participle ...]

4. B
This sentence is in the present tense, so "to find" is correct.

5. A
Always use the singular verb form for nouns like politics, wages, mathematics, innings, news, advice, summons, furniture, information, poetry, machinery, vacation, scenery etc.

6. A
Possessive pronouns ending in 's' take an apostrophe before the 's': one's; everyone's; somebody's, nobody else's, etc.

7. A
A bonus is an extra feature, so added is redundant.

8. D
When talking about something that didn't happen in the past, use the past perfect (if I had done).

9. C
"Lie" means to recline, and does not take an object. "Lay" means to place and does take an object. Peter lay the books on the table (the books are the direct object), or the telephone poles were lying on the road (no direct object).

10. A
Titles of short stories are enclosed in quotation marks.

11. C
No additional punctuation is required here.

12. B
Here the word "sale" is used as a "word" and not as a word in the sentence, so quotation marks are used.

13. C
If one of the subjects linked by "either," "or,""nor" or "neither" is in plural form, then the verb should also be in plural, and the verb should be close to the plural subject.

14. C
Titles of short stories are enclosed in quotation marks, and commas always go inside quotation marks.

15. B
"Ran well" is correct. "Ran good" is never correct.

16. D
Commas and periods always go inside quotation marks. Question marks that are part of a quote also go inside quotation marks; however, if the writer quotes a statement as part of a larger question, the question mark is placed after the quotation mark.

17. C
Conscientious is the correct spelling.

18. D
This is a declarative sentence.

19. C
A result is something that occurs at the end, so an 'end result' is redundant.

20. D
Both A and C are correct.

a. Their only employee with a nose ring is a young man named Daniel.

c. Their only employee is a young man with a nose ring named Daniel.

21. C
Use a singular verb with either, each, neither, everyone and many.

22. D
Leisure is the correct spelling.
23. C
Pigeon is the correct spelling.

24. D
Odyssey is the correct spelling.

25. C
Nouns like deer, sheep, swine, salmon etc can take a singular or plural verb depending if they are used in their singular or plural form.

26. A
Use an exclamation mark to end an exclamatory sentence, that is, at the end of a statement showing strong emotion.

27. D
Use an exclamation mark after an imperative sentence if the command is urgent and forceful.

28. D
Conclusive ADJECTIVE providing an end to something; decisive.

29. A
'He' is the simple subject of this sentence.

30. D
Deftly: VERB. Quick and skillful.

Section IV – Science

1. B
The only statement that is NOT true is, Phenotypes are inherited information.

2. D
All the above are true. Electrons play an essential role in electricity, magnetism, and thermal conductivity.

3. D
An idea concerning a phenomena and possible explanations for that phenomena is an hypothesis.

4. D
All of the above
a. Structures in a cell nucleus that carry genetic material.
b. Consist of one very long strand of DNA
c. Total 46 in a normal human cell.

5. B
One of the best known disorders that attack the immune system is HIV (the virus that causes AIDS).

6. D
The circulatory system disease that is one of the most frequent causes of death in North America is heart disease.

7. C
The plasma membrane or cell membrane protects the cell from outside forces. It consists of the lipid bilayer with embedded proteins.

8. A
The Strong Nuclear Force is an attractive force that binds protons and neutrons and maintains the structure of the nucleus, and the Weak Nuclear Force is responsible for the radioactive beta decay and other subatomic reactions.

9. D

Qualitative research deals with the quality, type or components of a group, substance, or mixture.

10. A

Adaptation is a trait that has evolved by natural selection.

11. A

A pH indicator measures hydrogen ions in a solution and show pH on a color scale.

12. B

The sun is the earth's primary source of energy.

13. B

The goal of quantitative research is to determine the relationship between one thing (an independent variable) and another (a dependent or outcome variable) in a population.

14. C

A base is any substance that can accept a hydrogen ion and can react with fats to form soaps.

15. D

The dominant gene controls the expression of a trait.

16. B

Plants and animals are Kingdoms. There are six recognized kingdoms: Animalia, Plantae, Protista, Fungi, Bacteria, and Archaea.

17. C

Organisms grouped into the **Protista** Kingdom include all unicellular organisms lacking a definite cellular arrangement such as **bacteria** and **algae.**

18. C

Indigestion is a common digestive affliction that most people suffer at one time or other.

19. D
Life functions are the biochemical and biophysical activities that all living systems must be able to carry out to maintain life.

20. C
Angina is frequently mistaken for a heart attack. Angina pectoris, commonly known as angina, is severe chest pain due to ischemia (a lack of blood, thus a lack of oxygen supply) of the heart muscle, generally due to obstruction or spasm of the coronary arteries (the heart's blood vessels). [24]

21. A
A collection of similar or like living entities. Class has the same meaning in biology as rank. Common classes or ranks include species, order, and phylum.

22. A
Fats stay in the stomach the longest.

23. A
A food web is a graphical description of feeding relationships among species in an ecological community.

Note: A food web differs from a food chain in that the latter shows only a portion of the food web involving a simple, linear series of species (e.g., predator, herbivore, plant) connected by feeding links. A food web aims to depict a more complete picture of the feeding relationships, and can be considered a bundle of many interconnected food chains occurring within the community.

24. D
A Punnett square resembles a game of tic-tac-toe, in which the genotypes of the parents gametes are entered first, so that subsequent combinations can be calculated.

25. D
All of these statements are true.

a. Prokaryotic cells include such organisms as E. coli and Streptococcus.

b. Prokaryotic cells lack internal membranes and organelles.

c. Prokaryotic cells break down food using cellular respiration and fermentation.

26. B
The process of converting observed phenomena into data is called Measurement.

27. A
The mass number of an atom is the total number of particles (protons and neutrons) that make it up.

28. B
Sublimation is the direct phase transition from solid to gas.

29. A
Exhalation is often accomplished by the abdominal muscles.

30. D
In Eukaryotic cells, the cell cycle is the cycle of events involving cell division, including mitosis, cytokinesis, and interphase.

31. D
All of the choices are correct.

a. The genetic makeup, as distinguished from the physical appearance, of an organism or a group of organisms.

b. The combination of alleles located on homologous chromosomes that determines a specific characteristic or trait.

c. Is the inheritable information carried by all living organisms.

32. D
The blood is the primarily oxygenated through the work of the respiratory system.

33. B
Ribonucleic acid (RNA) is a chain of nucleotides that play an important role in the creation of new proteins.

34. A
A practical test designed with the intention that its results will be relevant to a particular theory or set of theories is an experiment.

35. C
Covalent or ionic bonds are considered "strong bonds."

36. A
The process by which the immune system adapts over time to be more efficient in recognizing pathogens is known as acquired immunity.

37. D
An organ is a group of tissues that perform a specific function or group of functions.

38. D
Reliability refers to the measure of an experiment's ability to yield the same or compatible results in different clinical experiments or statistical trials.

39. C
Each chemical element has a unique atomic number representing the number of protons in its nucleus.

40. C
The immune system is the system that protects the body from disease and infection.

41. D
The plasma membrane surrounds the cell and functions as an interface between the living interior of the cell and the nonliving exterior. [19]

42. C
An organelle is a specialized subunit of a cell with a specific function.

43. A
A solution with a pH value of less than 7 is acid. A pH value of 7 is neutral.

44. B
A catalyst is never changed in a chemical reaction.

45. A
The prediction that an observed difference is due to chance alone and not due to a systematic cause; statistical analysis tested this hypothesis, and it is accepted or rejected is the **null hypothesis**.

46. C
In science and engineering, the Accuracy of a measurement system is the degree of closeness of measurements of a quantity to its actual (true) value.

47. B
High blood pressure is a more common name for the circulatory system disease known as hypertension. Hypertension (HTN) or high blood pressure is a cardiac chronic medical condition in which the systemic arterial blood pressure is elevated.

48. B
The range of a distribution is the difference between the maximum value and the minimum value.

Conclusion

C ONGRATULATIONS! You have made it this far because you have applied yourself diligently to practicing for the exam and no doubt improved your potential score considerably! Getting into a good school is a huge step in a journey that might be challenging at times but will be many times more rewarding and fulfilling. That is why being prepared is so important.

Study then Practice and then Succeed!

Good Luck!

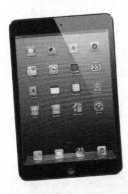

FREE Ebook Version

Go to http://tinyurl.com/m4abcfa

Register for Free Updates and More Practice Test Questions

Register your purchase at www.test-preparation.ca/register.html for fast and convenient access to updates, errata, free test tips and more practice test questions.

Complete Test Preparation

Inc. Scholarship

Enter to win an $800 Scholarship!

Write a 500 word essay on your best test preparation method, or, your best study skill!

https://www.test-preparation.ca/scholarship/

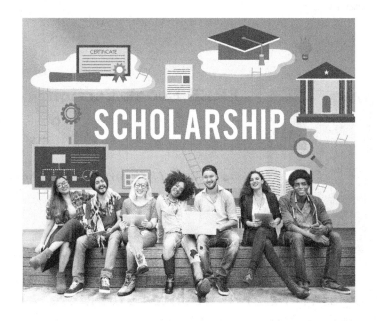

Made in the USA
Middletown, DE
04 December 2024

66071112R00099